# Mocked,
# Vilified,
## *and*
# Caricatured

A THEOLOGICAL RESPONSE FOR CLINICALLY
DEPRESSED AFRICAN-AMERICAN MEN FROM THE
PULPIT OF ONE OF AMERICA'S OLDEST BLACK
CHURCHES

# Mocked, Vilified, *and* Caricatured

A Theological Response for Clinically Depressed African-American Men from the Pulpit of One of America's Oldest Black Churches

By

## BRITT A. STARGHILL

This book was printed in the United States of America.

ISBN  0-9792953-4-3      978-0-9792953-4-8

Library of Congress Control Number:  2011939507


First Edition

This book can be purchased in bulk via the following distributors: Ingram, Baker & Taylor, Barnes & Noble, Amazon.com (U.S., U.K., & Canada) and Bertrams

Also available online at WWW.FULLSURFACEPUBLISHING.COM

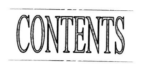

# CONTENTS

# ACKNOWLEDGEMENTS

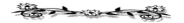

First, I would like to recognize my lovely wife, Catherine Frugé Starghill; my son, Britt II; my daughter, Brie Alexandra, who allowed me to be away to study, read, and write this book without ever complaining or grimacing; and my parents, Rev. Dr. Robert E. Starghill Sr. and Betty Jane Starghill, the greatest parents in this universe if you ask me. I would like to acknowledge and thank Ava Roland, my most trusted Administrative Assistant at Kaighn Avenue Baptist Church; Rev. Carla A. Jones, a reliable editor, reader and a very able minister at Kaighn Avenue Baptist Church; and the many great and laudable members of Kaighn Avenue Baptist Church of Camden, New Jersey, the oldest and greatest Baptist church in The State of New Jersey for which I have had the opportunity to serve as pastor over the last twelve years. Also, words cannot express the eternal gratefulness I have for Dr. James H. Evans, Dr. Gay Byron, and Dr. Barbara Moore, who are professors at Colgate Rochester Crozer Divinity School; they assisted me as invaluable readers, editors, and mentors for this project. Additionally, the Rev. Dr. John E. Duckworth, who is my cousin, friend, and brother and who pastors a great church in Michigan, is unmatched as a confidant. I cannot forget Marshall Mitchell and Tukumbo Adelakan, who are both great and intelligent friends that have encouraged me to continue to grow intellectually and culturally as well. Finally,

Robert E. Starghill, Jr., my brilliant brother, whose analysis of reality is always so pertinent. A large part of my desire and ability to do what I do comes from these particular friends, family members and pastors, as well as many other wonderful people that are in my life that give me confidence, encouragement, and the necessary resources to do my work, which I feel is God's work. This list of people doesn't cover everyone. The people in my life who have helped me along the way are really too many to mention yet too important for me to ever forget. Many pastors, professors, mentors, church members, and many other wonderful people who have all inspired me while encouraging, training, and correcting me all at the same time. Thank you and God bless you all! I relish and cherish you.

# ABSTRACT

Among other things, this thesis presents the idea that The Church can best respond to clinical depression among African-American men through education and ministry *that is focused on effective ministering and relevant real-time issues*. There is also a big need to enlighten the greater Christian community on many an issue concerning the collective position and condition of urban African-American men. I believe that enlightenment accompanied with education can foster awareness that promotes hope, new initiatives, social programs and resourceful ministries, and that local churches can help provide these in order to ameliorate and advocate change. My main objective here is to examine clinical depression among African-American men who are often unemployed, under-employed, disenfranchised, and projected in society as miscreants. In addition, I will argue that African-American men suffer disproportionately from clinical depression, which is often undiagnosed due to the economic pressures of poverty, class, racism, and the lack of communal and social support. To support this thesis, I will examine possible symptoms of clinical depression among African-American men in a local church in Camden, New Jersey. Additionally, I will propose a program of assistance in helping local churches become a catalyst for transformation for men suffering from clinical depression.

This discourse is written from the perspective that The Church, through the vernacular of prophetic ministry and transformation, should take the lead in raising the level of awareness within communities on the mental health condition of African-American men. The role of The Church is to act as a catalytic agent for transformation: to cultivate avenues for unconditional acceptance in order to foster a phenomenon wherein people's identities can be positively formulated and to push for the ideal of wholeness. I believe The Church can be a transformative institution capable of reaching these goals because its work is anchored in the belief that *all* are *Imago Dei*. (*Imago Dei*, translated from Latin, means that we are made in the image of God.) Moreover, the local church has the responsibility to minister to the *least* of us, for this is vital to the witness of Christianity.

In addition to addressing and acknowledging the severe need for awareness and information concerning African-American men suffering from undiagnosed clinical depression, I will also examine the structures that must be dealt with if clinical depression is to be sufficiently exculpated from the lives of African-American men. As I've said, the entire thesis is constructed within the framework of transformational leadership and prophetic ministry; both longstanding principal traditions of my alma mater Colgate Rochester Crozer Divinity School. These are also the personal traditions of this particular school's former professor Walter Rauschenbusch, who is one of my mentors and a former student of Rev. Dr. Martin Luther King, Jr., and my father and mentor Rev. Robert E. Starghill, Sr. who is a Baptist pastor in the City of Detroit's Southeast ghetto (by whom I was taught to champion the causes of the least, the lost, the marginalized, and the despised within society). I am wholeheartedly committed to those same traditions, thanks to them, and out of that commitment to foster justice and social equality this work emerges.

Chapter 1, entitled *WHAT IS GOING ON WITH AFRICAN-AMERICAN MEN?*, is an objective and reflective analysis of what scholars have written concerning the circumstances that describe the economic conditions in Camden, New Jersey, our 'scale' city of analysis for most of this book. This chapter describes Kaighn Avenue Baptist Church and some of the men who reside in the city and worship at the church who could be victims of clinical depression. The chapter cites some of the clinical traits that are symptoms of undiagnosed clinical depression within this particular community.

Chapter 2, *MAKING THE CASE THAT MANY AFRICAN-AMERICAN MEN ARE CLINICALLY DEPRESSED,* describes the different types of depression and gives descriptions of each type. Additionally, the issue of trauma is linked to depression as a causative effect for aberrant behavior within many African-American men. This chapter asserts that classifying psychic trauma as being a major root cause for clinical depression in African-American men is indeed a valid classification. This chapter also presents the argument that undiagnosed clinical depression *is* an overwhelming contributing factor to the rampant delinquency and crime that is plaguing our communities.

Chapter 3, *AMERICA'S OUTCASTS - AFRICAN-AMERICAN MEN: MOCKED, VILIFIED, AND HUMILIATED* gives a description of the various consequences that black men face because of undiagnosed depression. Furthermore, this chapter illustrates how the consequences of trauma are exhibited within African-American men's lives.

Chapter 4, *A THEOLOGICAL REFLECTION FOR AFRICAN-AMERICAN MEN,* is constructed within a theological perspective to describe the condition and social position of African-American men today. This theological reflection contextualizes and subscribes the biblical text of the Gerasene demoniac (demon possession) in

Mark 5:1-20 to African-American men today, as part of the explanation for our collective marginalization and outcast status. Additionally, this chapter raises the issue of "the War on Drugs" as actually being a war on poor African-American men who are exploited, demonized, and suffering from social alienation today and being heavily incarcerated in prisons and institutions.

Chapter 5 is entitled *DEVELOPING A MODEL FOR LIBERATION AND TRANSFORMATION*. This chapter aptly describes a tried model of ministering to clinically depressed men in the setting of Kaighn Avenue Baptist Church that can and should be used nationally and possibly even internationally. This ministry model is specifically designed for African-American men who live with certain stresses and pressures to which many African-American men in urban areas are most vulnerable. The focus of this chapter is to create a tool to assist, foster, and promote ministry for the specific life needs of African-American men in distressed urban areas in the United States.

It is my greatest hope that the information contained in this work will be of some aid to African-American men everywhere who are or may be suffering from clinical depression. I am a big believer that *faith without works is dead*, so we ourselves must first *believe* and then *work* to find the answers to the problems that too many African-Americans suffer from. Work is contribution, and we all have to contribute if we are to find those answers and then solve our problems. Let us first believe and understand, and then do work!

# Chapter 1

## WHAT'S GOING ON WITH AFRICAN-AMERICAN MEN?
### A Small Scale Historical Perspective of the Big Picture

### The Migration History of My Hometown of Camden, New Jersey

Camden, New Jersey might seem to be a perfect place to test this hypothesis on clinical depression being heavily present amongst African-American men. Listed as one of the twenty-four "cities past the point of no return," Camden could legitimately be described as one of the places in this country that lends credence to the notion that many African-American men are quintessentially in a form of inner city or 'under-class' degradation and are in the perfect position to suffer with clinical depression.[1] Due to economic and social exclusion and discrimination against them, African-American men in most urban areas are an essential means to engage in a definitive study of some of the root causes and symptoms of clinical depression.

Camden had an overall poverty rate of 44% in 1995 - the highest rate in the country - and the lowest wealth index in relation to its suburbs and surrounding jurisdictions.[2] Through a congruence of factors, Camden is a microcosm of how

---

[1] Gillette, Jr., Howard. *Camden After The Fall: Decline and Renewal in a Post-Industrial City* (Philadelphia, PA: Philadelphia Press, 2005) Pg. 8.
[2] Ibid.

the ill effects of urban unemployment, associated with antisocial behavior, and poverty have contributed to a legacy for those who are unable or unwilling to leave the city for new opportunities while living in conditions of deteriorating homes, shrinking employment opportunities, and inferior social services. Additionally, Camden offers the special advantage of not being so large as to escape comprehensive/thorough examination. Nearly universally impoverished, it offers a case study of how an entire population that is comprised of African-American men, not just some of its constituent elements, operates within a climate of crushing austerity, thus bringing to the fore the central dynamics of just how a typical group of African-American men deal with poverty/disenfranchisement within the context of urban poverty. In short, while Camden offers a small stage scenario, all the major issues associated with the descent of the classic blue-collar city appear in recognizable form and in comprehensible fashion.

Camden originally developed largely as an extension of Philadelphia, which during the colonial period was the leading city on the North American continent. Camden's incorporation in 1828 did not remove it from the larger city's sphere; Philadelphia remained its closest urban nexus neighbor directly across the Delaware River and continued to exercise influence by using Camden in the pursuit of business and personal interest.[3] The city began to acquire standing on its own in 1834, when the Camden and Amboy Railroad, then the longest rail line in the country, made Camden its terminus. In testimony to its growing importance, the town became the county seat in 1844.[4] Although it remained in Philadelphia's shadow up through the Civil War era, Camden's peaceful growth attracted both immigrant work and the capital to establish its own industrial base. Camden

---

[3] Ibid. Pgs. 18-38.
[4] Ibid. Gillette

became home to manufacturing plants that produced carriages, woolen goods, and lumber, and to Richard Esterbrook's Steel Pen Company. In 1891, the modest canning business Joseph Campbell had started in 1869 incorporated as Campbell Soup. Eight years later the New York Ship Company opened shipping yards in Camden, which soon employed as many as 5,000 workers. In 1901, Eldridge Johnson, who had begun work on a "talking machine" two years earlier formed the Victor Talking Company.[5] Other smaller but important manufacturing firms joined these three emerging giants to produce everything from fountain pens to cigars. By 1909, Camden's Board of Trade could assert "the city has within these ten bright and busy years thrown off the shackles inspired by a fear of being so near to a metropolitan city." A 1917 report listed 365 industries in Camden, employing 51,000 people.[6]

By 1920, Camden's population exceeded 100,000 for the first time, ranking the city 58th in population nationally, just behind New Bedford, Trenton, and Nashville and ahead of Lowell, Wilmington and Forth Worth. By 1924, anticipating the opening of the new forty million dollar bridge which would be named after Benjamin Franklin, it was extended two miles in length and rose 385 feet above the high tide mark.[7] Later on in 1954, the Chamber of Commerce journal *Camden First* proclaimed on its cover, "Camden is a growing metropolitan city. No longer a satellite city, she stands on her own feet, her eyes to the stars. She sees great development ahead, she is all but ready."[8] An advertisement in the same journal saw Camden as a "second Brooklyn". By 1935, the *Philadelphia Evening Bulletin* was forced to admit that Camden had created its own tributaries and was the

---

[5] Ibid.
[6] Ibid. Gillette
[7] Ibid.
[8] Ibid.

beneficiary of "a very considerable amount of trade which does not cross the river."[9]

By then Camden had started to show signs of being affected by the rest of the nation's deep economic depression. Right after the mid-1930's, the city's business owners became so economically bankrupt that the city had to pay its workers in scrip. Nonetheless, a directory of Camden enterprises in 1937 fully suggested the full strength of the city's underlying industrial foundation. The city's big three manufacturers continue to employ large numbers of residents: Campbell Soup (5,600) New York Ship Company (5,522) and RCA Victor (13,030).[10] Other well-known industries as well as smaller companies, ranging from metalwork to shipbuilding, textiles, and soap making businesses, complemented the giants. Edna Martin recalls, "With so many factories ringing the city, most people walked to work and downtown.[11] Every morning there would be crowds on the streets. One would find children walking to school, people working and hurrying to their respective places of employment. Different starting times meant different bursts of sound."[12]

Work remained plentiful for those arriving in Camden all the way up to the early 1950's. Camden's vital entrepreneurial activity was manifested within a series of commercial corridors, most notably along its major commercial corridors of Broadway, Haddon, Westfield and Kaighn streets.[13] On these streets, one would find movie theaters, doctors, dentists and lawyer's offices mixed with a host of commercial and retail services. In addition, neighborhood commercial corridors

---

[9] Ibid.
[10] Ibid.
[11] Ibid. Gillette
[12] Ibid.
[13] Ibid.

emerged to serve specific ethnic constituencies. In the years from 1931 to 1947, some of the most tumultuous years encompassing not just the depression but a world war, the city thrived and more than half the foundational businesses of the city remained in the same hands without closing. Where businesses did change hands they still remained similar in kind; mainly family-owned operations serving the local community.

The City of Camden survived the most difficult of times and emerged virtually intact beyond both the Great Depression and World War II.[14] Such continuities should not be oversimplified or overemphasized, however; in an era where jobs carried no tenure and few public forms of insurance existed to counter the unexpected changes of either the marketplace or the life course, working people had to rely on others in times of difficulty. For the most part, that meant turning to those of the same ethnicity. Germans, Irish, Poles, Eastern European Jews, Lithuanians, and Italians may have worked in different establishments but they clustered together in homes located close to churches or synagogues where services often were conducted in their native language.[15] They formed their own communal associations that would provide different services for them in times of emergency. Therefore, ethnic and communal ties were reinforced through these elaborate social structures that also strengthened their sense of belonging both to a particular neighborhood and to a larger ethic group. Nearly every ethnic group made it a point to organize themselves in the various communities throughout the city during this period, and those same networks still exist in Camden to this very day.

---

[14] Ibid.
[15] Ibid. Gillette

## The Presence of African-American Congregations in Camden and the Socio-economic Destruction of the City

During the first half of the 20th century, African-Americans remained primarily parochial and isolated from the other communities in Camden that were comprised of other ethnicities. As I've said, each unit of the larger urban fabric held strongly unto itself, recognizing other units but keeping a certain distance, but this phenomenon was compounded and exercised with extra zeal when it came to African-American communities. Each ethnicity had its own distinct neighborhood: Whitman Park was called "Polaktown" where the Polish-Americans lived; North Camden was "Irishtown"; North Camden and "Germantown" is what later came to be known as the Cramer Hill section; and a mixed section called "color town" or "dago town" - in South Camden in the industrial district was where "colored" people otherwise known as African-American and Latin Americans clustered.[16] (African-Americans and Latin Americans have surprisingly longstanding parallels in housing options in Camden.)

The African-American presence and contributions in Camden stretch all the way back to the 1830's. The South Camden neighborhood of Fettersville was home to the very first black churches; Macedonia AME (1832) Union AME (1855) and Kaighn Avenue Baptist (which started as a prayer meeting in 1838 and organized as a church in 1856).[17] Other organizations pertinent to the African-American community were the West Jersey Orphanage for Colored Children and the John Greenleaf Whittier Colored School for Girls and Boys. The black migration to the city increased before and during World War II, with an additional community

---

[16] Ibid.
[17] Ibid.

formed in the Centerville section of the city between Whitman Park and South Camden.[18] In addition to the presence of several prominent black churches, an expansive swimming pool drew African-Americans from around the region as well as from the immediate residential area.

So although ostensibly a part of a somewhat integrated North, Camden was nearly as segregated as if the city had been located below the Mason-Dixon Line. Segregation started early in any black child's life in Camden. Even though they lived close to the Starr School for Girls and the Liberty School for Boys in South Camden, these were "whites only" educational institutions, thereby forcing African-American students to walk additional blocks to the all-black Whittier, despite where they lived. African-Americans customarily traveled on the back of the bus. When they had the chance to see a performance at the Stanley Theater downtown, they were required to sit together in the upper balcony. African-Americans were systemically and methodically marginalized and segregated throughout the city; Campbell Soup was one of the largest employers in the city at that time and though it had a good record of employing blacks the company did design separate restrooms by race in its new 1941 plant.[19] So like other black communities in the U.S. that were forced to turn inward due to external discrimination, the African-American community in Camden did develop its own array of specialized services, including doctors' offices, lawyers, barbershops, funeral homes and real estate services.[20]

Industrial work for African-Americans was especially difficult to obtain on a sustained basis and was subject to a number of perils. Although RCA did not hire

---

[18] Ibid. Gillette
[19] Ibid.
[20] Ibid.

many black workers, those lucky enough to hold long term positions found themselves at the bottom of the scale, in terms of both pay and desirability. Many African-American families were prompted to find other ways to secure cash. Some of the ways in which money was secured was the illegal numbers operations called "policy", the predecessor to lottery, which flourished in the city through the 1930's into the 1950's.[21] While Italians dominated this business in South Camden, such type operations extended throughout the city. South Camden, the African-American area, was widely recognized as the headquarters of this activity.

What is the context of the social, economic, and cultural elements which contributed to the dramatic changes in the city? Furthermore, what created the environment for the social turmoil that accelerated a process of white migration out of the city? In my mind, several convergent patterns stand out. First, black and white settlement patterns between 1940 and 1970 mirror each other.[22] That is, approximately as many whites left the city in each decade as African-Americans arrived, offering sure confirmation of the importance of the riots and associated social turmoil in accelerating a process of white migration out of the city. Secondly, manufacturing losses relate to some white departures but do not appear to have solely driven the exodus process that incurred. Most striking, in fact, is how well manufacturing employment held up during the immediate postwar period through 1960. Camden listed slightly more industrial jobs in 1960 than in 1948, paralleling total employment growth in the city.[23]

Over the next decade though, the pace of both job losses and white departures accelerated. Between 1960 and 1967, industrial employment fell sharply by 12,000

---

[21] Ibid. Gillette
[22] Ibid.
[23] Ibid.

jobs.[24] The city lost another 7,000 industrial positions in the following three years alone, the result in part of New York Ship's closure, one of the largest employers in the city at that time. In a single decade Camden's manufacturing base declined by 48%.[25] In fact, the 1970's marked the onset of what Barry Bluestone and Bennett Harrison characterized in their classic 1981 study as "the de-industrialization of America". Skilled positions represented over half of the losses in jobs in Camden, and it would not have been surprising, given both the more cosmopolitan ties of these workers and the shift in employment by RCA, in particular, to the suburbs, to see this group add to the stream of white flight-migration. African-Americans, whose presence was always limited in heavy industry, were less affected, but as their numbers continued to grow they competed more with whites for housing. Workers congregating in older and thus more affordable housing located near the city's industrial core had reason enough to leave when they lost jobs. Pressure to sell their homes gave them one more excuse to leave when they lost jobs, however attached they might have been to their old neighborhood. During the 1960's another 28,000 whites left Camden. Now indisputably, economic change was contributing to the metropolitan area's demographic shift, even before the civil disturbances of 1971.[26]

Industrial employment continued to decline in the 1970's, though not as rapidly as white flight rose. By the end of the decade, two features stood out: Camden could no longer be considered a manufacturing center, nor was it a predominantly white working class city. For the first time, whites no longer constituted a majority of Camden but rather just over 30% of the city's total population.[27] In this light,

---

[24] Ibid.
[25] Ibid.
[26] Ibid. Gillette
[27] Ibid.

Camden's civil disturbances assumed particular importance as a convenient trope, giving power and specificity to Camden's transformation. To the degree that racial and economic change were conflated in the public mind, subsequent reports of rising crime and social disorder, or what the Manhattan Institute's Fred Siegel calls " rolling riots," sealed the city's reputation as an undesirable place. From there, it was not a great distance to denigration for the people, African-Americans, who were behind and burdened with the legacy of disinvestment, marginalization, and redlining as being responsible for their misfortune. It is worth examining the process that leads to the crystallization of such conclusions about this post - industrial city, not unlike many a black city in the U.S. whereby these same kinds of conditions created fertile ground for African-American men to suffer from clinical depression.

As aforementioned, for years African-Americans and Puerto Ricans had been confined to the oldest and least desirable housing stock in the city. Housing conditions in distinctly black neighborhoods were inferior to those outside of it. As whites began to move out, absentee landlords (who highly elevated the rent, I might add) often rented out homes.[28] After the 1950 U.S. Census reported that 5,000 of Camden's 38,000 homes lacked indoor toilets, the Courier-Post, the local paper, commented editorially that there were more people than it liked to admit "living under conditions like those under which million of Asiatics live, amid filth, over- crowding and all the factors that breed disease and crime."[29] During this period of white flight, economic discrimination, and unfair housing practices, specious arguments were advanced that the victims of these practices, African-Americans, were victims of their own laziness, indifference, etc. Civil rights

---

[28] Ibid. Pgs. 39-62. Gillette
[29] Ibid.

organizations were often protesting and doing demonstration to advance the rights of the African-American community. By the late 1960's, militant black power advocates began to champion for more extreme measures to gain civil rights for African-Americans within the city.[30] Political unrest and socio-economic tensions began to rise exponentially until several civil rebellions culminated.

In 1973 the economic and social conditions that Camden's African-Americans lived under became extremely dire, and federal funds for urban renewal programs that had offered some hope were effectively terminated.[31] Other categorical grant programs favoring cities had been reduced in favor of revenue sharing with states. Across the country, cities like Camden faced deep budgetary shortfalls. In Camden, not only were revenues well short of meeting essential needs, the rate of serious crimes had climbed to the second highest in the country. The mayor of the city at that time, Mayor Angelo Errichetti's description of his city on his first day of work as mayor was graphic: "It looked like the Vietcong bombed us (Camden) to get even."[32] The prideful city of Camden...was now a rat-infested skeleton of yesterday, a visible obscenity of urban decay...the years of neglect, slumlord exploitation, tenant abuse, government bungling, indecision and short-sighted policy had transformed the city's housing, business and industrial stock into a ravaged, rat-infested cancer on a sick, old industrial city.[33]

During the mid-late 1970's, the tax base of the city continued to fall, while huge deficits began to really wreak havoc and destroy the city and its majority African-American population. The precipitous decline in the city also undermined the

---

[30] Ibid.
[31] Ibid.
[32] Ibid. Pg. 89. Gillette
[33] Ibid.

political process.[34] In 1960, about 1/3 of the county voted, however, by 1980 only 16% casted votes.[35] As long as the Great Society persisted, social programs could be tapped to supplement the city's declining revenues. Thus, as the federal funding to urban areas was abandoned during the Reagan presidential years, Camden really became the place of the lame, poor, and downtrodden. Simultaneously, inner cities all across the nation became symbols of despair, high unemployment, crime infestation, drug trafficking, drug addictions and centers of urban decay. Whereby, as the rest of South Jersey, the suburbs, gained political strength, wealth, and population etc., Camden became both poorer and weaker politically and economically.[36]

Finally, by 1980, the day of the Great Society federal funding was over. The country seemed ready to let cities like Camden shift for themselves but without the political strength it once had, Camden itself was in no position to dictate the terms of political rewards. "I tried to use mirrors to give the image of strength of the city," Culnan, one of the reporters of the Courier-Post quoted Errichetti, a former mayor of the city as saying. "But the smart people could see the real numbers...Camden's no longer the hub of South Jersey or the county; it's just a joke." Fast forward to March of 1991- Camden had lost two of its last largest employers, with Campbell Soup retaining its world headquarters in the city but closing its last processing plant and consequently laying off an additional 900 workers.[37] During the same time period RCA Victor ownership was bought out by the Martin-Marietta Company, later to become a part of the multi-national conglomerate General Electric, which quickly moved the company outside of the

---

[34] Ibid.
[35] Ibid.
[36] Ibid. Gillette
[37] Ibid.

city altogether while closing its plant within the city.[38] The departure of the big manufacturing plants triggered the demise or exodus of the smaller stores, several banks, and other businesses that relied on the wages paid by the large employers for their revenue. It has been estimated that Camden lost 75% of its business establishments from 1960 to 1970 alone.[39] Camden had at its apex well over 115,000 people; today the city has fewer than 90,000 people and many of them are children in disproportionally poor and single parent households.[40]

To make plain some of the causes and consequences of such occurrences, in 1945 St. Clair Drake and Horace Cayton's classic study *Black Metropolis* was published.[41] Drake and Cayton first examined black progress in employment, housing, and social integration using census, survey, and archival data. Their analysis clearly revealed the existence of a color line that effectively blocked blacks' occupational, residential, and social mobility. They demonstrated that any assumption about urban blacks duplicating the immigrant experience had to confront the issue of race.[42] The fact is the disappearance of work and the consequences of that disappearance for both social and cultural life are the central problems for most African-American men in urban areas or inner city ghettos. To acknowledge the fact that most ghettos are created by lack of opportunity and joblessness is to also acknowledge that those who live in those conditions are highly likely to be clinically depressed from the aftermath. It is the argument of this study that the combination of systemic racial practices such as restrictive covenants, redlining by banks and insurance companies, zoning, panic peddling by

---

[38] Ibid.
[39] Ibid.
[40] Ibid.
[41] Wilson, William Julius. *When Work Disappears: The World of the New Urban Poor* (New York: Vintage Books, 1996) Pgs. 18-33.
[42] Ibid. Gillette

real estate agents, and the creation of massive public housing created the milieu for social isolation of individual African-American men from their families and communities, and thereby are heavy contributing factors for disadvantage and denial of opportunity, for African-American men.

Currently, Kaighn Avenue Baptist is located in the south central district of the city, called "Gateway" on Ninth and Kaighn Avenues. The congregation is the oldest African-American Baptist Church in the state of New Jersey. Though some of the men in Kaighn's congregation are from nearby suburbs and are very educated, well-employed, with high paying jobs, nonetheless, the congregation serves many residents who are suffering from sundry constraints and very high joblessness. These constraints, combined with restricted opportunities in the larger society, lead to behaviors and attitudes that are found more frequently in ghetto neighborhoods or very poor African-American communities than within neighborhoods that feature even modest levels of poverty and local employment. Ghetto-related behavior and attitudes often reinforce the economic marginality of the residents of jobless ghettos. I use the term "ghetto-related" as opposed to "ghetto-specific" so as to make the following point: Although many of the behaviors to be described and analyzed are rooted in circumstances that are unique to inner city men, they are not fairly widespread in the larger society. In other words, these behaviors are not unique to ghettos, as the term "ghetto-specific" would imply; rather they occur with greater frequency in ghettos, where African-American men often reside.

What is also ghetto-related is heavy unemployment and bad underfunded educational forums. The unemployment rate for African-American men in Camden is over 50%, and there are few legitimate employment opportunities as well as inadequate job networks and poor schools.[43] Graduation rates are below 50% in two of the four high schools in the city, Camden High and Woodrow Wilson.[44] These two schools are ranked the lowest two schools in the state, ranking 314 and 315.[45] Indeed, poor schools also do lead to disappearance of work and low expectations for the future of any given community. That is, where jobs are scarce, people rarely, if ever, have opportunities to help their friends and neighbors find jobs and there exists a disruptive or degraded "school life" to prepare youngsters for eventual participation in the workforce. In this kind of culture some young men lose their feelings of connectedness to work in the formal economy. Indeed in this context, they no longer expect work to be a regular and regulating force in their lives. In the case of some of the men in the congregation of Kaighn Avenue, many of them have grown up in environments that lack the idealized work experience. In many households where the men were reared, few people in the house worked. Additionally some of the men have very little education outside of high school, therefore having low or no skills for higher paying jobs. These circumstances also increase the likelihood that some men will rely on illegitimate sources of income, thereby further weakening their attachment to a legitimate labor market.

Camden is a city were 65% of the home loans were subprime in 2007; only 3.5% of the citizens have bachelor's degrees; and less than 25% of the population has a $9^{th}$ grade education.[46] In the context of poverty and joblessness, William Julius Wilson, a sociologist at Harvard University writes that, "Unstable work and low income, I would hypothesize, will lower one's perceived self-efficacy."[47] A recent

---

[43] U.S. Census Bureau News. *U.S Department of Commerce* - Washington, D. C. printed February 14, 2008.
[44] Jill P. Capuzzo. *Formula for Success*. New Jersey Magazine, Sept. 2008. Vol. no. 9, Pgs. 72-75.
[45] Ibid.
[46] U. S. Census Bureau News. *U. S. Department of Commerce* - Washington D.C. - printed February 14, 2008.
[47] Wilson, William Julius. *When Work Disappears: The World of The New Urban Poor* (New York: Vintage Books, 1996) Pg. 76.

study on the negative affects of adverse economics on mental health and even parental behavior, based on data from both black and white inner city parents in Philadelphia, provides some support for this hypothesis. The study reported that mounting economic pressures, caused by unstable work and low income, created feelings of emotional depression and thereby tended to lower the parents' sense of efficacy in terms of what they believed to be their influence over their children and on their children's environment.[48] Wilson further argues "I would therefore expect lower levels of perceived self-efficacy in ghetto neighborhoods - which feature underemployment, unemployment, and labor force dropouts, weak marriages and single parent households - than in less impoverished neighborhoods.[49] Wilson argues that the longer the joblessness persists, the more likely these self-doubts will take root within one's self-consciousness. This is true within the context of a city like Camden plagued by economic marginality one could easily suffer from much lower levels of self-efficacy, where strong feelings of marginality could easily grow into clinical depression.

## How This All Ties In:
## The Root of Clinical Depression for Many African-American Men

The symptoms of clinical depression in the context of men who are poor and reside in inner cities like Camden are usually not recognized as clinical depression but instead are typically described as aberrant and deviant behavior. Therefore, to detect African-American men who are suffering from clinical depression we would have to analyze the life-threatening affects and side effects of clinic depression when it's not acknowledged nor diagnosed in men who are most likely to be

---

[48] Ibid.
[49] Ibid.

unaware of the chronic disease. Some of these symptoms include but are not limited to suicide; crime; various addictions; overeating; high blood pressure; overworking; juvenile detention; prison relapse; sexual promiscuity; shattered relationships; divorce; excessive materialism; job loss; hopelessness and listlessness.[50] Researchers and mental health professionals, including pastors, must look closely at how violence operates not only in the form of criminal behavior, but also as domestic and child abuse. Violence in many African-American communities expresses some of the frustration and hopelessness felt by many who are clinically depressed, and homicide often becomes a byproduct of suicidal impulses.

The roots of depression are constantly feeling powerless and helpless; feeling a loss of control of one's life; feeling a sense of distrust of everything and often everyone; feeling there is something intrinsically wrong with yourself, and not being able to distinguish what causes anguish and anxiety. Furthermore, one who suffers from clinical depression is in a perpetual state of feeling vulnerable and sad. People who are suffering from depression are not able to sustain "normal" relationships at work, home, nor various communities. People sense an overwhelming "hollowness" in their lives, which disturbs one's self-identity. In this state of vexation one is unable to control their reality.

Our sorrow and helplessness make us turn away from our pain. The pain congeals and clinical depression sets in. When it comes to depression, many individuals in the African-American community do not understand the dynamics, the warning signs, and the available treatment. For decades, depression has been

---

[50] Williams, Terrie M. *Black Pain: It Just Looks Like We're Not Hurting* (New York: Scribner Press, 2008). Pgs. 28-30.

considered a stigma or a crippling label in many social circles. Many people jump to pin the label "crazy" on anyone who is suffering from clinical depression. What many people don't realize is that depression is a medical ailment that can be explained in terms similar to your achy joints or seasonal allergies, and whether it's genetic, situational, or spontaneous, depression is as common as a stuffy nose.[51]

The Church and community must realize that a person doesn't choose to become depressed any more than a person chooses to catch a cold. It happens! What we have to do as a church/community is move past the prevailing ignorance that has held us back in understanding, treating, and preventing clinical depression among African-American men. We have to encourage discussions within our circles on African-American men's depression. The Church must become open-minded in order to begin to address this issue.

---

[51] Ibid.

# Chapter 2

## MAKING THE CASE THAT MANY AFRICAN-AMERICAN MEN ARE CLINICALLY DEPRESSED

### Understanding the Crisis with African-American Men

### Analyzing Education; Employment & Unemployment; Delinquency & Crime; Substance Abuse; Unwed Teenage Parenthood; Homicide & Suicide

Cornel West, in his book *Race Matters*, argues that there are structural constraints on the life chances of African-Americans (men) which involve a subtle historical and sociological analysis of slavery, Jim Crowism, job and residential discrimination, skewed unemployment rates, inadequate health care and poor education that perpetuate the plight of African-Americans at the bottom rung of the social ladder. Alternatively, there are those who stress that behavioral impediments on black upward mobility are the cause for lack of upward mobility. The advocates of the belief that African-Americans (men) are socially immobile usually focus on a waning Protestant ethic – lack of hard work, lack of deferred gratification, absence of frugality, and exhibiting privation in responsibility - as the explanation for much of African-American's want of progress.[52] West also suggests that these two arguments are not expansive enough to engage the "real issue": the nihilistic

---

[52] West, Cornel. *Race Matters* (Boston: Beacon Press, 1993) Pgs. 11-20.

threat to the very existence of African-Americans, especially African-American men. Cornel West avowals that:

Nihilism is to be understood here not as a philosophic doctrine that there are no rational lived experience of coping with a life of horrifying meaninglessness, hopelessness, and (most important) lovelessness. The frightening result is a numbing detachment from others and a self-destructive disposition toward the world. Life breeds a coldhearted, mean-spirited outlook that destroys both the individual and others. [53]

The nihilism that West cites as a loss of hope and absence of meaning in his book becomes a self-fulfilling prophecy; without hope there can be no future. Without meaning, there can be no real construction of a fruitful life for many African-American men. West also argues that the affects of the culture of "random nows," of fortuitous and fleeting moments preoccupied with getting everything *"now"* [54] are very apparent. This lifestyle of acquiring pleasure, property, and prestige at all cost has had a profound affect on African-Americans. Perhaps this is what the rapper Curtis "50 Cent" Jackson means in his hit movie and top-selling music project entitled *Get Rich or Die Trying.* This particular hip-hop mogul's "gangsta" game face almost cost him his life, which is not at all uncommon when it comes to many young black men in his field. In an interview in America Magazine, Jackson says:

I spent the majority of my life being angry. Anger is my most comfortable feeling. If I'm upset or my feelings are hurt, I become angry; if I become angry; if I'm confused, I become angry. Like if one of my "homies" (friends) got shot or stabbed at the club. You're upset because you feel for him, but instead of going somewhere and crying about it, you get angry. Then, after you

---

[53] Ibid.
[54] Ibid.

respond, you change to having jitters about law enforcement finding out about what you just did.[55]

Unfortunately, there is a zeitgeist of this kind of thinking that has created a "gangsta" culture in America, particularly in urban ghettos where hyper-materialism is projected to be everything. Moreover, this milieu has perpetuated the degradation and oppression of many African-American men who are desperate for identity, meaning, and self-worth amid the privation of inner cities. In a postmodern culture where markets are all about selling things, it is extremely dangerous when the gangster rap culture promulgates images of African-American men (images embraced by many African-American men and syndicated by the media throughout the world) as gangsters/thugs, belligerent, and wanton. This culture engulfs many of us, both male and female - yet its impact on African-American men is most devastating; resulting in despair, being dispirited and internalizing feelings of listlessness. Many African-American men see themselves as being hapless in a society where everything that one should be able to obtain only a few actually have access to obtaining and thus have internalized the belief that they can rarely attain The American Dream due to prejudice, racism, and lack of gainful employment. It is out of this marinating, desperate thinking and feeling that this form of popularized gangsterism was spawned. Now, to say that it has become most problematic for our communities is a gigantic understatement; it has actually become one of the leading tangible causative factors for African-American males being considered as an endangered species.

An endangered species is, according to Webster's Dictionary, "a class of individuals having common attributes and designated by a common name...

---

[55] Williams, Terrie M. *Black Pain: It Just Looks Like We're Not Hurting* (New York: Scribner Books, 2008) Pg. 19.

{which is} in danger or peril of probable harm or loss."[56] This description applies, in a metaphorical sense, to the current situation of African-American men in many urban areas of America. Many African-American men are living in and around urban areas and are either miseducated by the educational system, mishandled by the criminal justice system, mislabeled by the mental health system, and/or mistreated by the social welfare system. All the major institutions of American society have failed to respond appropriately and effectively to African-American men's multiple needs and problems. Consequently, many African-American men are unequivocally living unenviable lives of almost total rejection. Many African-American men undeniably live dejected lives that are counter-affluent to most people in the dominant society. Thus, most African-American men are indeed seen as miscreants, misfits and criminals, even within their own neighborhoods and communities.

As a result of all this, African-American men that predominantly live in urban inner cities, working class suburbs, and in small towns all over America are also increasingly subjected to the adversarial scrutiny of social scientists, educators, politicians, and especially the mass media. Oftentimes these men are not only living below the poverty line but also are living underneath society's radar screen; working "under the table" (avoiding federal and state tax collection) is a frequently used term in and by members of the African-American community denoting working and earning wages illegitimately or illegally. Unfortunately, when some of them find out that these type of marginal survival methods are hard to sustain, they basically give up and that's why many African-American men can be found loitering on street corners, playing sports on playgrounds or on school lots during

---

[56] Gibbs, Jewelle. et.al. *Young Black and Male in America: An Endangered Species* (Dover, Massachusetts: Auburn House Publishing Company, 1988) Pgs. 1-5.

workday work hours, selling drugs in alleys, and talking/arguing in front of convenient stores and local bars. The media regularly refers to African-American men using a variety of specious labels and ways such as "underclass", the "inner city/urban population", "the "unemployed", "welfare pimps", and even more pejorative terms that are ever increasing, signifying negativity about African-American men. Derisively, too many African-American men seem to internalize this kind of nomenclature and refer to themselves (on an everyday basis) in similar negative ways as well. These terms are: "thug", "hustler", "pimp", "killer" and an unending list of other terms that assist in labeling themselves negatively. Labels are powerful clues to the ways in which groups are perceived, valued and plausibly treated, but labels cannot convey the true feelings of frustration, humiliation, and anger of these black men who experience daily traumatic experiences that cause frustration, humiliation, and disillusionment.

Additionally, African-American men are portrayed by the mass media in limited, often compromised roles, most often being deviant, dangerous, and dysfunctional. The constant barrage of predominantly disturbing images and roles predictably contributes to the public's negative stereotyping of African-American men presumably as young, hostile, and impulsive when in fact they are traumatized. Furthermore, even the supposedly, positive images of African-American athletes and entertainers are projected as animal-like, infantilized, hostile, aggressive, hyper-violent, flamboyantly materialistic, sensual, along with being politically and culturally obviated. Evidently, there is a message saying: If they entertain you, enjoy them; if they serve you, patronize them; if they threaten you, then avoid them.[57] Psychologist Jewelle Taylor Gibbs asserts in her book entitled *Young Black*

---

[57] Ibid.

*and Male in America: An Endangered Species* that African-American men are negatively stereotyped thoroughly. She identifies African-American men as having been caricatured in society as the five "D's": Dumb, Deprived, Dangerous, Deviant, and Disturbed.[58] She argues that because of this popularized caricature there is no room in the larger social picture for comprehension, caring, or compassion for the plight of African-American men. Whereas there are many social indicators pertaining to African-American men that provide a merited hypothesis that many African-American men are suffering from clinical depression, she argues in the book that there are several specific social indicators that put African-American men at great risk. These indicators are: Education, Employment/Unemployment, Delinquency & Crime, Substance Abuse, Unwed Teenage Parenthood, and Homicide & Suicide.[59] Let us analyze these particular indications further.

## Education

Statistics on the general educational attainment of African-Americans have been improving over the past 25 years.[60] For example, the proportion of high school dropouts among black youth in the 14-24 age group steadily declined from 23.8% in 1960 to 13.2% in 1984, and for 16-17 year olds, from 22.3% to 5.2% in the same period.[61] In more recent years the gap between black and white overall dropout rates in the high school age group has indeed shortened, except for the disproportionately high rates among inner city black youth. In most urban areas, the high school dropout rate is 50%. In some places, like Detroit for example, it's

---

[58] Ibid. Pg. 3.
[59] Ibid. Pgs. 6-15.
[60] Ibid. Pg. 6.
[61] Ibid.

as low as 25.6%, which is still much too high.[62] Even before getting to and through high school though, there are surveys that estimate that more than 20% of black male adolescents in the 12-17 age group were unable to read at the 4th grade level.[63] Some of those within that group would undoubtedly go on to graduate but many will not; in 1980, statistics indicated that 21% of all 18 and 19 year old black males and 25% of all 20 and 21 year old black males had neither completed nor were presently enrolled in high school.[64] Statistical figures do not reveal the number of African-American young men with high school diplomas who are functionally illiterate or barely able to fill out a job application, which is prevalent enough, so though things have somewhat improved statistically for blacks in terms of general educational attainment, we have to wonder: How many African-American men with high school diplomas are currently functioning without the necessary skills for most entry-level jobs, apprenticeship programs, military service, or postsecondary education?[65] All indications point to that number being much higher than it should be as well.

Still, poor and mediocre academic performance along with dropping out of high school remains a big problem for black male youth. While reasons for dropping out of high school are varied, a recent Urban League study pointed out that many African-American male teenagers leave school because of family economic problems, academic difficulties, disciplinary problems, and learning disabilities that are sometimes attributable to coming from disadvantaged households and impoverished communities. Moreover, inner city students are confronted with

[62] U. S. Census Bureau News. U. S. Department of Commerce - Washington, D.C. printed February 14, 2008.
[63] Gibbs, Jewelle. et. al. *Young Black and Male in America: An Endangered Species* (Dover, Massachusetts: Auburn House Publishing Company) Pgs. 6-31.
[64] Ibid.
[65] Ibid.

nearly insurmountable barriers to learning and achievement in schools that are characterized by poorly prepared teachers, inadequate educational facilities, low teacher expectations, ineffective administrators, rampant misappropriations and chronic violence.

The clear cut consequences of black teenagers academically performing poorly and dropping out of school or only obtaining meaningless and near-worthless high school diplomas based on an expectation of "social promotion" are higher rates of unemployment, fewer job options, greater welfare dependency, and long-range limitations on their social and economic viability. I submit that these various factors contribute to African-Americans being stuck on the bottom economically in this country while immigration, downsizing, and outsourcing continue to exacerbate the decreasing job market.

### Employment/Unemployment

Unemployment among African-American men is nearly 3 times higher than it is for white American men.[66] In many urban areas, the unemployment rate for African-American men is at least 50%.[67] The unemployment rate for African-American men has consistently been higher than that of African-American women by a ratio of two to one for nearly forty years.[68] Unemployment among African-American young men was 34% - twice the rate of 17.4% among all teenagers.[69] Unemployment statistics obviously reflect the labor force participation rates of African-American men, which have fallen dramatically since 1960. At that time,

---

[66] Ibid. Gibbs, Jewell. et al.
[67] Ibid.
[68] Ibid.
[69] Ibid.

## MAKING THE CASE THAT MANY AFRICAN-AMERICAN MEN ARE CLINICALLY DEPRESSED

82% of African-American men ages 20-24 participated in the labor force, but in 1980 only 73.5% of this group participated.[70] However, by 1980 less than 1/3 were able to find jobs. In 1983, African-American high school dropouts were twice as likely to be unemployed, with only 26% of them in the labor force.[71] That trend has continued and today, African-American men are increasingly unable to find jobs and many of them that are in poverty, as I've mentioned, are often unprepared to assume more gainful employment, which is increasingly required in a global society where competitive, highly technological skills are the norm. Moreover, recent studies have indicated that chronically unemployed men constitute a disproportionably high percentage of those workers who become "discouraged" and completely drop out of the job seeker's market. Without gainful employment, African-American men are progressively more vulnerable to participate in the alternative economy of the urban ghetto - that is, the illegal system of bartering stolen goods, drugs, gambling and other criminal activity.

The reality of a rapidly declining group of African-American men who are unemployed, unemployable, and who are being socialized towards nonproductive lifestyles on the streets is majorly implicated in creating conditions for suffering from clinical depression. The question could be raised, how can the average person subjected to these variables not be at some point driven "crazy", made "sad" or "blue", "humiliated" or as the medical terminology describes it, clinically depressed? Living with the desperation and anguish of this kind of existence has created a crisis for many African-American men who reside in urban areas. As aforementioned, as an unconscious alternative, droves of African-American men are gravitating towards images and lifestyles that depict themselves as ruthless

---

[70] Ibid.
[71] Ibid.

thugs, violent drug dealers, sexual predators, and absent fathers; outlaws on the outskirts of society. A prominent question rises within this context: Why are African-American men, who have labored in the cotton fields, worked in the coal mines, built federal buildings, constructed state and federal roads, been steel workers and worked in various factories - all of a sudden now unwanted and unemployable in American industry today? These are relevant issues that point toward the malaise affecting African-American men, particularly in inner cities.

## Delinquency and Crime

The culmination of African-American men suffering from disproportional unemployment and lack of educational advantage contributes to increased crime, arrests, and incarceration. It is not difficult to acknowledge that crime is often a residual when people are not able to function in a society. African-American men are arrested more frequently than whites for robbery, rape, homicides, and aggravated assaults.[72] Moreover, African-American men are more likely to be arrested for other violent personal crimes, disorderly conduct, sexual misbehavior, and handling stolen property. FBI reports compiled from the mid 1970's indicate that African-American men accounted for nearly 1/3 of all arrests.[73] During the same period, over half the juvenile arrests for the most violent crimes were among African-American youth. Those numbers, though high then, have increased dramatically. The "class" of inner city African-American men who viciously burglarized outside of their own communities are now increasingly brutalizing their own neighborhoods, stores, and homes, vandalizing schools with violent acts, while being projected in the media as culprits in society for terrorizing the greater

---

[72] Ibid. Pgs. 8-39.
[73] Ibid. Gibbs, Jewelle. et al.

community as well. Therefore, these images of African-American men are promulgated throughout the world, while simultaneously vilifying African-American men as being the nation's foremost criminals. Not surprisingly, this allegation is synchronized with the notion that the judicial system is "too light" on crime.[74]

Despite the bias of statistics and other ways of compiling data, it is particularly disturbing to note that African-American men are significantly more likely than any other ethnic group to be incarcerated in federal and state prisons and facilities and are represented in much higher numbers in prisons, jails and other correctional institutions. The crucial question is: Who are the real culprits in these statistics - those who are being observed (African-American men and boys) or the circumstances and conditions that produce this travesty? Why are so many African-American men in prison? What is causing this pandemic in America, where so many African-American people, usually poor and illiterate, are in prison and involved in the penal system? What is the proper solution to alleviate this crisis?

## Substance Abuse

Although a number of recent studies for the CDC (Center for Disease Control) have indicated that in early adolescence the overall rate of drug and alcohol use is actually lower among African-American youth than white youth, the rates of heroin and cocaine use, including the recent derivative for poor people called "crack", are disproportionately high among older African-American teenagers.[75]

---

[74] Ibid.
[75] Ibid. Gibbs, Jewelle. et al.

## MAKING THE CASE THAT MANY AFRICAN-AMERICAN MEN ARE CLINICALLY DEPRESSED

Reliable estimates of drug use in this population are difficult to obtain due to sampling problems and other methodological issues, but too many studies of selected samples of young black men within major metropolitan areas suggest high lifetime usage rates for these drugs. For example, a study in Harlem studying African-American men in the mid 1970's found that heroin and cocaine rates were 3 times higher than reported by a national sample of selective service registrants.[76]

The issue is not simply illegality or immorality. Society's concern should be focused on the damage these young people are inflicting upon themselves physically, psychologically, and socially.[77] Among many other things, drug use among African-American men is highly correlated to low school achievement, delinquency, and accidental deaths.[78] Furthermore, drug addiction for the inner city black male demographic almost inevitably involves theft, drug sale and use, and even hustling sex in order to get high: crime. Drug addiction among African-American men substantially increases the risk of arrest and imprisonment, physical and mental illness, and death by overdosing.[79] Young addicts lose interest in both school and work and gradually deteriorate so much that getting high becomes the major motivation of each day; eventually they become walking zombies, worthless to themselves, their families and their communities. This type of self-destruction from drugs has implications of something that is entrenched and furtively ticking away, with the insidious danger of a time bomb, to explode within many African-American men. Consequently, what social forces are involved in shaping the vulnerabilities of these men? What are the risk factors that promulgate their great

---

[76] Ibid.
[77] Ibid.
[78] Wilson, William Julius. *When Work Disappears: The World of The New Urban Poor* (New York: Vintage Books, 1996) Pgs. 51-75.
[79] Ibid. Wilson

need to create an escape from reality? What is latently inherent within drug addiction that makes many African-American men so susceptible? These are salient questions that need to be asked and engaged by the entire community; government, public servants, The Church, and every individual.

## Unwed Teenage Parenthood

During the 1980's, the Guttmacher Institute published a startling report that said the pregnancy rate for American teenagers from the ages of 15-19 years old were the highest of all industrialized nations at 96 per 1,000 pregnancies per year. In 1980, America was also the only country where the pregnancy rate was increasing more rapidly among white adolescent females than their black female counterparts but now out-of-wedlock pregnancy has become an entrenched problem in the African-American community as well.[80] In 2000 for example, nearly 1 in 10 African-American teenage females gave birth compared to one in twenty-five white females.[81] Pregnancy rates are now twice as high among African-Americans as white Americans (163 per 1,000 vs. 83 per 1,000) and surveys suggest that 70% of all African-American children are now born out of wedlock. [82]

These offspring from these pregnancies, that are really the children of children, and particularly the boys, have a great propensity to have profound physical and psychosocial consequences. The mothers of these boys are more likely to drop out of high school, more likely to go on welfare, and more likely to experience complications in pregnancy. Babies born to teenage mothers are more likely to

---

[80] Ibid. Pg. 13.
[81] Ibid.
[82] Kunjufu, Jawanza. *State of Emergency: We Must Save African-American Males* (Chicago: African-American Images, 2001) Pg. 149.

have low birth weights and other prenatal and postnatal problems and are usually less healthy, less academically successful in school, more likely to grow up in a single parent welfare-dependent family, and more likely than children born to adults to become single parents themselves.[83] They are also much more likely to experience abuse and neglect as either givers or takers of it.

The effects of premature fatherhood on the youthful male partner of these teenage relationships have only recently been of interest to researchers but several studies have found that, compared with their peers who have not fathered children, these young men are more likely to attain lower educational levels and lower occupational status, to have larger families, and to experience unstable marriages.[84]

## Homicide and Suicide

The final and most alarming social indicator is the increase in mortality rates among young African-American men, particularly from homicides and suicides. Homicide is now the leading cause of death for African-American teenagers.[85] In 1960, the homicide rate for African-American men was 46.4 per 100,000. This rate increased through the next two decades, reaching a peak of 102.5 per 100,000 in 1970 and then declining to 61.5 per 100,000 in 1984. However, the current rate is still 33% higher than it was twenty-five years ago, a level unacceptable in a civilized society. An African-American man has a one in twenty-one chance of being murdered before he reaches the age of 25. In 2005 alone, more than 2,000

---

[83]Gibbs, Jewelle. et. al. *Young Black and Male in America: An Endangered Species* (Dover, Massachusetts: Auburn House Publishing Company) Pgs. 6-40.
[84] Ibid.
[85] Thompson, Rondel. et al. *The State of Black America 2006* (New York: National Urban League Press, 2006) Pgs. 46-57.

# MAKING THE CASE THAT MANY AFRICAN-AMERICAN MEN ARE CLINICALLY DEPRESSED

African-American men were murdered - over 90% of them by other African-American men.[86]

While Euro-American youth die primarily from accidents, African-American youth die primarily from homicide. These homicide statistics are a direct result of gangs and drug trafficking in the inner cities, where gangbangers and drug dealers employ violence with impunity in cities like Philadelphia, Detroit, Camden, Newark, Chicago, and Washington, D.C., where they often use semi and fully automatic machine guns to protect their turf and terrorize their neighborhoods, oftentimes killing innocent bystanders. There is often a culture of excessive violence, the brandishing of high-powered weapons, and a pervasive disregard for life, which creates a profound alienation away from normalcy and community.

In 1960, the suicide rate for African-American males was 4.1 per 100,000. Since then, African-American men have death rates that are at least twice as high as those of women for suicide, cirrhosis of the liver, and homicide.[87] From 1980 to 2005, the suicide rate for African-American young men (ages 15-19) increased by 146%.[88] (Among African-American young men ages 15-19, firearms were used for 72% of suicides while strangulation was used in 20% of suicides.[89]) For African-American men, especially in urban areas, the consequences of abusing alcohol and drugs appear graver when comparing suicide statistics with European-American men and women or African-American women, since these sicknesses are connected to suicide. Young African-American men are more likely to commit

---

[86] Ibid.

[87] *Souls of Black Men: African-American Men Discuss Mental Health.* Centers for Disease Control and Prevention. 1998b. Suicide Among Black Youths-United States, 1980-1985. Atlanta, GA: US Department of Health and Human Services Centers for Disease Control and Prevention.

[88] Ibid.

[89] Ibid., GA: US Department of Health and Human Services Centers for Disease Control and Prevention.

suicide after an altercation or perceived victimization by institutional authorities such as police, criminal justice system, school officials, landlords or welfare department.[90] Among African-Americans, especially men, the possibility of "being someone" or making a significant contribution to society and attaining basic respect and self-esteem is always a goal but seldom a reality, predisposing them to suicidal and homicidal acts of self-destruction.

Although suicide rates among African-American men are still lower than European-Americans in every age group, studies suggest that the figures would be much higher if many causes of death among African-American men in general were reported as symptoms of clinical depression; if some of the gang violence, deliberate drug overdoses, victim-precipitated homicides, deaths from AIDS, cases of cirrhosis of the liver/alcoholism, uncontrolled diabetes, strokes, heart attacks, and fatal altercations with police were counted as suicides. Clearly these factors and conditions contribute to feelings of hopelessness and thereby increase African-American men's vulnerabilities to (and participation in) suicidal behavior.[91] William Julius Wilson, in his book *When Work Disappears* argues that when neighborhoods are plagued by high levels of joblessness people in those communities are more likely to be faced with neighborhood problems like crime, gang violence, and drug trafficking, which in turn causes family breakups and other problems in the organizational family life as well.[92] I concur with that assessment. The trauma that is so apparent from these events in the lives of many African-American men produces lasting affects on the psyche, which are rarely acknowledged or treated. It becomes imperative to analyze the culmination of the

---

[90] Ibid.
[91] Ibid.
[92] Wilson, William Julius. *When Work Disappears: The World of the New Urban Poor* (New York: Vintage Books, 1996) Pg. 21.

brutal events and stress with which many African-Americans are constantly confronted when the outcome is the dire reality we are faced with today in our communities. The truth is that many psychiatrists believe that many men in the inner city are suffering from post-traumatic stress disorders.[93]

In summary, these six social indicators - education, unemployment, delinquency and crime, drug abuse, teenage parenthood, and mortality rates from homicide and suicide - are bellwethers of the serious problems facing and experienced by many African-American men. Each of these problems contributes to a larger problem that is both psychological and social, and the outcomes and consequences are all inextricably connected to clinical depression.[94] I submit that many African-American men are quietly suffering from the residuals of various traumas from their personal experiences and thus are suffering from undiagnosed clinical depression. The traumatic experiences that many African-Americans men have endured in America make this argument substantive. This argument of trauma is substantiated by the brutal treatment of African-American men not only in historical times but in modern times as well. The combination of the cruelty of slavery, lynching, unremitting disenfranchisement, economic redlining, chronic unemployment, relentless police brutality, legal executions, and ghetto homicides have undoubtedly produced an unparalleled psychic trauma for African-American men in the United States.

---

[93] Ibid. Pg. 105.
[94] Ibid.

# Chapter 3

## AMERICA'S OUTCASTS:
## MOCKED, VILIFIED, AND HUMILIATED

### The Many Consequences of Clinical Depression & Trauma

### Analyzing Types of Depression; Clinical Depression Symptoms; Psychic Trauma & Trauma's Effects

"Slavery: …that slow poison, which is daily contaminating the minds and morals of our people. Every gentleman here is born a petty tyrant. Practiced in acts of despotism and cruelty, we become callous to the dictates of humanity, and all the finer feelings of the soul. Taught to regard a part of our own species in the most abject and contemptible degree below us, we lose that idea of the dignity of man, which the hand of nature had implanted in us, for great & useful purpose."

*George Mason, July 1773*
*Virginia Constitutional Convention* [95]

Terrie M. Williams, a licensed clinical social worker, in her book *Black Pain – It Just Looks Like We're Not Hurting* writes:

For black men, the never-ending quest to be a man, and society's putting down of that manhood, is an open wound that never closes. Some men find ways to provide themselves with a sense of worth that does not come directly from the outside world; for many others this task is harder.

---

[95] Blackmon, Douglas A. *Slavery by Another Name: The Re-Enslavement of Black Americans from the Civil War to World War II* (New York: Double Day Broadway Publishing Group, 2008)

Unable to shake the idea that they are less-than in the eyes of the culture, they begin to evolve defense mechanisms that sow the seeds of depression.[96]

Many African-American men feel like racism, unemployment, under-employment, and social vilification have stripped them of their power. Some black men react to this feeling either by overachieving at the expense of their emotional well-being or underachieving at the expense of their material and emotional well-being. Both responses still leave African-American men open to stifling self-doubt and low self-esteem and fearful of their own potential weakness. Over time, emotionally denying oneself and the shame that comes from having to constantly prove that the culture's racist attitudes are wrong can lead a man to feel secretly like he *is* less than a man.

The official number today tells us that at least 7% of African-American men experience severe depression during their lifetime.[97] We have no numbers to tell us how many more are typically plagued by low-level ongoing depression (*dysthymia*).[98] For many years, depression was seen as a women's disease. Depression carried the stigma of being "feminine".[99] However, generally, depression in men is much higher than ever imagined but goes largely unacknowledged and undiagnosed both by men that suffer from it and those who surround them. All the while, the impact of this hidden depression is enormous in America.[100] One of the reasons that depression in men is not easily detected is because men suffer from depression differently than women. Women are more likely to talk about things that disturb them, while men are trained to keep more in

---

[96] Williams, Terrie M. *Black Pain: It Just Looks Like We're Not Hurting* (New York: Scriber, 2008) Pg. 81.
[97] Ibid. Pgs. 77-125.
[98] Ibid.
[99] Ibid.
[100] Ibid.

and not talk about things that concern them.[101] Many men are content to quietly suffer from depression; therefore we must distinguish the current understanding of depression and the three most common types of depressive disorders so that we recognize the symptoms when we see them. However, within these distinctive types of depression there are variations in the number of symptoms, their severity, and persistence.[102] Depressive disorders come in different forms, just as it is the case with other illnesses such as heart disease. A depressive disorder is an illness that involves the body, mood, and thoughts. It affects the way a person eats and sleeps, the way one feels about oneself, and the way one thinks about things. A depressive disorder is not the same as temporarily passing through a "blue" mood and it is not a sign of personal weakness or a condition that can be willed or wished away. People with a depressive illness cannot merely "pull themselves together" and get better. Without treatment, symptoms can be reoccurring and can last for weeks, months, or even years. Appropriate treatment, however, can help most people who suffer from depression.[103]

## Types of Depression

**Major depression** is manifested by a combination of symptoms that interfere with the ability to work, study, sleep, eat, and enjoy once pleasurable activities. Such a disabling episode of depression may occur only once but more commonly occurs several times in a lifetime. A less severe type of depression, **dysthymia,** involves long term, chronic symptoms that do not disable, but keep one from functioning well or from feeling good. Many people with dysthymia also

---

[101] Real, Terrence. *I Don't Want To Talk About It: Overcoming the Secret Legacy of Male Depression.* (New York: Scribner Books, 1997) Pgs. 21-66.
[102] Ibid.
[103] Ibid.

experience major depressive episodes at some time in their lives.[104] Another type is **bipolar disorder,** also called manic-depressive illness. Bipolar disorder is not nearly as prevalent as other forms of depressive disorders. Bipolar disorder is characterized by cycling mood: severe highs (mania) and severe lows (depression). Sometimes the mood switches are dramatic and rapid, but most often they are gradual. When in the depressive cycle, an individual can have any or all of the symptoms of a depressive disorder. When in the manic cycle, the individual may be overactive, over-talkative, and have a great deal of energy. Mania often affects thinking, judgment, and social behavior in many ways that cause serious problems and oftentimes embarrassment. For example, the individual in a manic phase may feel elated, full of grand schemes that might range from unwise business decisions to romantic sprees. Mania, left untreated, may worsen to a psychotic state.

## Clinical Depression Symptoms

It's important to remember that not everyone who is depressed experiences every symptom. Some experience a few symptoms, others experience many. The severity of symptoms of depression varies with individuals and also varies over time.[105] The limited scope here is just to concentrate on clinical depression and how its symptoms are pervasive among African-American men in inner cities. Here's a list of many of those symptoms:

| Persistent sad, anxious, or "empty" mood |
| Feelings of hopelessness, pessimism |
| Feelings of guilt, worthlessness, helplessness |

---

[104] *Souls of Black Men: African-American Men Discuss Mental Health.* Center of Disease Control and Prevention, 1998. Suicide Among Black Youth-United States, 1980-1985. Atlanta, GA: US Department of Health and Human Services for Disease Control and Prevention. Pgs. 2-5.
[105] Ibid. Center of Disease Control and Prevention.

| |
|---|
| Loss of interest or pleasure in hobbies and activities that were once enjoyed, including sex |
| Decreased energy, fatigue, being "slowed down" |
| Difficulty concentrating, remembering, making decisions |
| Insomnia, early-morning awakening, or oversleeping |
| Appetite and/or weight loss or overeating and weight gain |
| Thoughts of death or suicide; suicide attempts |
| Restlessness, irritability |
| Persistent physical symptoms that do not respond to treatment, such as headaches, digestive disorders, and chronic pain |
| Grandiosity/ extremely materialistic |
| Hyper-violence & hyper-masculinity |
| Homicidal/gangbanging/proliferation and obsession of guns |
| Obsession with sexuality/pornography |
| Standing on corners, listlessness |
| Alcoholism/drug addictions |
| Fantasizing about death/ attraction to certain types of Rap/ lyrics |
| Need for control - particularly over women/lovers |
| Unusual aggressiveness - anti-authority |

[106]

According to statistics, only 9% of men have suffered from or will ever suffer from depression - but statistics may not be completely accurate.[107] As I've pointed out, statistics and most written works on the subject only reveal a portion of the larger community impact. Although I have found several books that address female depression, to my knowledge there is only one other book that specifically focuses on African-American men's depression exclusively. The book is *Black Men and Depression* by a journalist, John Head. Hence, the question of being able to acknowledge the severity of depression among African-American men is not even

[106] Ibid.
[107] Ibid.

on the radar of the world! What a catastrophe that African-American men are not even considered to be diagnosable, while persistently being reported in the news as the primary harrowing agents of America's cities.

In Terrence Real's insightful book on men's depression *I Don't Want to Talk About It: Overcoming the Secret Legacy of Male Depression,* he argues, as I do, that African-American men are suffering from depression at rates far higher than what statistics show. Specifically, in the African-American community, the homicidal rates, drugs, diseases that are controllable yet fatal, perpetual violence, the disproportional imprisonment, and suicidal choices are incalculable. The truths behind much of these activities are the symptoms of clinical depression, though most people have not identified it this way. In some cases there are diagnosis issues, as some African-American men are suffering from bipolar disorder and others are in a state of dysthymia. The truth is, many of these African-American men are not just ruthless criminals, lawless felons, and shiftless villains; rather they are undiagnosed victims of society suffering from clinical depression, and the pain, exclusion, and ignorance limits the prognosis. As I've said, many African-American men suffering with mental anguish don't feel good about themselves, thinking they're flawed or seeing themselves as worthless outcasts. In fact, when men do not feel they can measure up to what is purported to be "real" manhood (having a "good" job and being able to adequately provide for their families) this causes extreme trauma for many men.[108]

One of the ironies concerning men's depression is that the very forces that help create it, keep men from seeing it. Men are not supposed to be vulnerable. Pain is

---

[108] *Souls of Black Men: African-American Men Discuss Mental Health.* Center of Disease Control and Prevention. 1998b. Suicide Among Black Youth-United States, 1980-1985. Atlanta, GA: US Department of Health and Human Services Center for Disease Control and Prevention. Pgs. 2-5.

something we are supposed to rise above. Sadly, in our culture, a man who has been brought down by it will most likely see himself as shameful. Hidden depression drives several of the problems we think of as typical to urban African-American men. The kind of depression that most African-American men suffer is not referenced in most of the literature about the disorder. The guidebook for diagnosis used by most clinicians throughout the country is the American Psychiatric Association's *Diagnostic and Statistical Manual of Mental Disorders* (DSM IV) which labels a person as having a clinical depression only if he or she shows, for a duration of at least two weeks, signs of either feeling sad, "down," "blue," or having a decreased interest in pleasurable activities, including sex.[109] So since males are trained to keep more in and not talk about things that concern them, men are more likely to suffer from covert depression while women are likely to suffer from overt depression. [110] Generally, men suffer from depression that is brought on by failed expectations and disconnections from their culture and family. Some call this "masked depression" or underlying character logical depression.[111]

The condition described in the DSM IV is the classic form of depression most of us think of. Although many men may be reluctant to admit that they are suffering from overt depression, the disorder itself has been recognized since ancient times. As early as the 4th century B.C., Hippocrates, the European "father of medicine," reported a condition that had symptoms that included "sleeplessness, irritability, despondency, restlessness, and possibly an aversion to food" - a description of overt depression easily recognizable today.[112] Hippocrates saw the malady as caused by an imbalance of the black bile, one of the four humors, and he therefore

[109] Real, Terrence. *I Do Not Want To Talk About It: Overcoming the Secret Legacy Of Male Depression* (New York: Scribner, 1997) Pgs. 21-41.
[110] Ibid. Pgs. 38-41.
[111] Ibid.
[112] Ibid.

named the disease "the black bile," which in Greek reads *melanae chole*, or melancholia.[113] Researcher Martin Opler observed this depression type as far back as 1974: "Masked depression is one of the most prevalent disorders in modern American society, yet it is perhaps the most neglected category in psychiatric literature." Moreover, I submit that masked depression is the most prevalent disorder in modern American society, particularly today. Overt depression in men seems to be overlooked in society and covert depression in men has been rendered all but invisible among white men. Thus, it is almost never mentioned as a diagnosis for African-American men. [114]

As a black man and as the pastor of an African-American church, I agree with Martin Opler that the masked depression that is often covertly noticed in white men becomes conspicuous in many African-American men in urban areas due to the many common symptoms exhibited throughout most urban ghettos. Thus, what he describes as covert depression I assert is undiagnosed clinical depression often masked as nihilism or ennui. For covertly (undiagnosed) depressed African-American men, what lies at the center of the depression? In most cases for men that suffer from covert depression, the answer, as aforementioned, is trauma. For some men, underlying emotional injuries are blatant and extreme. For others, they are seemingly mild, even ordinary. In both instances, the covertly depressed has tendencies to damage or sever emotional connections between themselves and others. No matter if the injuries are publicly known or unknown, depressed men carry inside of them a hurt, bewildered little boy whom they scarcely know how to

---

[113] Ibid.
[114] Ibid. Pgs. 38-41. Real

care for. Befittingly, Henry David Thoreau once wrote: "The mass of men lead lives of quiet desperation."[115] This is doubly true for African-American men.

I am fully convinced that the issue that is at the center of covert depression/masked depression/clinical depression is shame or trauma. While depression may carry some sense of stigma for all people, the disapprobation attached to this disease is particularly acute for men. The very definition of manhood lies in "standing up" to the discomfort and pain. I believe that many African-American men run from their internal distress, interpreting masculinity as being "strong" or "never vulnerable to circumstances". This is what Terrance Real describes in many men who are suffering from clinical depression when he writes, "All too often, denial is equated with tenacity - under the bludgeoning of chance my head is bloody, but unbowed."[116] Terrance Real argues that this attitude compounds a depressed man's condition, so that he gets depressed about being depressed, ashamed about feeling ashamed. Because of the stigma attached to depression, men often allow their pain to burrow deeper and further from view. Many men are ashamed of their feelings and refuse help because their perception is that they are suffering from a "wimp disease", as it has been called, and are unaware that it can potentially kill them in various ways.[117] Case in point: Men are 4 times more likely than women to take their own lives.[118] Men take "being strong" and "making it" personal, and African-American men struggle with the improbability of "making it" in a society that overwhelmingly views them as

---

[115] Ibid.
[116] Pgs. 38-41. Real
[117] Ibid.
[118] Ibid.

second class and thus as a group are indeed definitely more predisposed to acts of self-destruction.[119]

## Psychic Trauma

Research on the biology of trauma is beginning to teach us that even apparently mild childhood injuries can produce lasting physiological change. Moreover, the harmful effects of trauma often go unrecognized and consequently, undiagnosed. As a culture historically dominated by male values, we have always tended, and still tend, to deny vulnerability, and consequently, to deny the existence of trauma. Sigmund Freud was the first psychotherapist on record to document patients' reports of childhood trauma and sexual abuse. In one of the most famous mistakes of the 20th century, Freud decided that female patients, often daughters of friends and colleagues, were lying about their traumatic experiences; he emphatically denied the possibility that the presumably decent men he knew could do the things these young women reported.[120] Consequently, he did what many have done throughout history when faced with trauma survivors: he disbelieved and blamed the victims.

The issue of trauma did not surface again until tens of thousands of "shell-shocked" solders forced psychologists to consider the topic once during World War I. At first, we tried to deny the reality of psychological injury, blaming physical injury instead. (The term "shell-shock" derives from the mistaken theory that the distress occurs as a result of a concussion from explosives.) When it

[119] *Souls of Black Men: African-American Men Discuss Mental Health.* Center of Disease Control and Prevention. 1998b. Suicide Among Black Youth-United States, 1980-1985. Atlanta, GA: US Department of Health and Human Services Centers for Disease Control and Prevention.
[120] Ibid. Pgs. 87-112.

became clear that American soldiers were not physically but emotionally overwhelmed, they themselves were blamed for it. The public rhetoric shifted from the language of medicine to the language of moral weakness; shell-shocked soldiers lacked "fiber", it was said. They were considered frail malingerers or, more bluntly, cowards. The new medical specialty field of psychiatry, brought out of relative obscurity into the mainstream because of the need to treat those combat veterans, dressed up essentially the same sentiments in technical terms; offering up the picture of the "neurotically susceptible" and "infantile" male.[121] Not until the grassroots movement of Vietnam veterans forced the medical establishment to stop blaming the victim, did we as a culture acknowledge for the first time that any man, no matter how "high" or "low", could be emotionally overwhelmed if subjected to enough stress. Out of this a new diagnosis, Posttraumatic Stress Disorder, usually referred to as PTSD, was born.[122]

## Trauma's Effects

What is the impact of 200 years of U.S. slavery, coupled with oppression, and high unemployment, underemployment, being psychologically castrated - rendered impotent in the economic, political, and social arenas that whites have historically dominated? African-American men learned a long time ago that the classic American virtues of thrift, perseverance and hard work did not give them the same tangible rewards that are accrued to European American men. Furthermore, in order to begin to understand the magnitude of this legacy on contemporary African-American men, it is vitally important to examine the diagnostic characteristics of trauma. What are the effects of trauma on human beings? What

---

[121] Ibid. Real
[122] Ibid.

does trauma look like? How does the trauma manifest itself? What is known about trauma that makes it probable that significant numbers of African-American men warrant a diagnosis of PTSD? The *Diagnostic Statistical Manual of Mental Disorders IV, Revised,* helps clinicians with making accurate diagnoses by describing symptoms and features of disorders and reporting the conditions that may eventually give rise to mental illnesses. However, it is not necessary for an individual to show evidence of all of the listed symptoms to warrant being diagnosed with specific illnesses. The following chart lists some of the conditions which give rise to mental and/or emotional trauma that justify the diagnosis of PTSD:

| |
|---|
| Intense psychological distress at exposure to internal or external cues that symbolize or resemble an aspect of the traumatic event |
| Physiological reactivity on exposure to internal or external cues |
| Marked diminished interest or participation in significant activities |
| Feeling of detachment or estrangement from others |
| Restricted range of affect |
| Sense of foreshortened future (in other words, does not expect to have a career, marriage, children or normal life span) |
| Difficulty falling or staying asleep |
| Irritability or outburst of anger |
| Difficulty concentrating |

African-American men and the American culture have defined the totality of manhood in terms familiar to European American men - as breadwinners, providers, procreators, and protectors. Unlike Euro-American men, African-

American men have not had consistent access to the means with which to fulfill their dreams of masculinity and success in this culture and many have become frustrated, angry, embittered, alienated, and impatient. Some have learned to permanently mistrust the words and action of the dominant culture. The stress of enduring the denial of systemic disenfranchisement, and social normalcy results in trauma, the source of clinical depression. [123]

The book *Traumatic Stress: The Effects of Overwhelming Experience on Mind, Body, and Society* states that PTSD is a result of a failure of time to heal all wounds. Additionally, the book asserts that the core issue is the inability to integrate the reality of particular experiences and the resulting repetitive replaying of the trauma in images, behaviors, feelings, physiological states, and interpersonal relationships. Therefore, in dealing with traumatized people, it is critical to identify and examine where they have become "stuck" as a way of acknowledging their trauma and which specific traumatic event(s) they have built into their secondary psychic elaborations and set up effective cultural defense mechanisms. Oftentimes culture is the only defense of dealing with trauma. Culture is supposed to render life predictable. When the cultural defense mechanisms are lost, individuals are left on their own to try and achieve emotional control. So when traumas that occur within the context of social upheavals (such as unemployment, being in protracted periods of being unemployed, underemployment, and marginalization) they do cause lasting psychic trauma to those affected. When one internalizes the effects of being powerless or feeling absolutely worthless, emotions will promote a profound discontinuity from society whereby anxiety and panic are exaggerated. This is

---

[123] Ibid.

trauma; emotional shock that accompanies extreme distressing experiences, which often causes long lasting psychological effects.[124]

## The Consequences of Trauma

Physiologically, there is a drastic change in the body of a person who suffers from depression. When trauma is not dealt with and handled properly, it can create emotional problems including anxiety, irritability, fatigue and depression. The brain will begin to produce a hormone called cortisol.[125]Cortisol is an important hormone that circulates in the body all the time, increasing and decreasing within each 24 hour period. This particular hormone does some very useful things: it mobilizes fat for use as energy; it is an anti-inflammatory agent; it is involved in the functioning of the liver; and it may increase the sensitivity to detection of threats.[126] Under stress, there is an increase in circulating cortisol and it turns out that prolonged elevation of cortisol is bad for a person. It can be destructive to the immune system; causing chronic fatigue syndrome and undesirable changes in various areas of the brain that are involved in memory.[127] So although science has well established the life changing impact of trauma, science is still exploring the ways in which traumatic experiences actually affect the physiological development of the brain in the long term. Psychologists are increasingly interested in how trauma alters the activity of neurotransmitters and hormones.[128] However, it is unequivocally clear that trauma leaves lasting effects on the brain. [129] So although the brain and body are both remarkable malleable, they both yearn for an existence

---

[124] Ibid.
[125] Real, Terrence. *I Do Not Want To Talk About It: Overcoming The Secret Legacy Of Male Depression* (New York: Scribner, 1997) Pgs. 38-41.
[126] Ibid.
[127] Gilbert, Paul. *Overcoming Depression: Step-By-Step to Gaining Control Over Depression* 2nd Ed. (New York: Oxford Press, 1997) Pg. 3.
[128] Pgs. 3-5. Gilbert
[129] Ibid.

that is comfortable, balanced, loving, and happy. Nonetheless, if the impact of trauma is present but not treated and promptly addressed - the probability of complete healing is weakened. The more time passes between trauma and intervention, the greater its hold on the person and the more difficult it becomes to reverse its effects. Thus, the trauma that African-American men suffer socially, economically, and mentally never gets recognized as a cause for mental illness or as having any responsibility for economic conditions within urban areas throughout the United States.[130]

The over-presence of two of the most common symptoms of PTSD, hyper-arousal and dissociation, can rightly be considered as strong evidence that many African-American men are suffering from clinical depression. It is my argument that these two categories for PTSD are the most descriptive symptoms of clinical depression within many African-American men. Hyper-arousal is also known as hyper-vigilance. A hyper-aroused person is always looking out for danger and quick to react when any danger is sensed - often perceiving real danger where none exists. In this state, something as benign as direct eye contact, a hand on the shoulder, stepping on someone's sneakers or boots, or a simple criticism is blown far out of proportion, and the person reacts.[131] The other aspect of this is the hyper-vigilant man, who is in a constant "fight or flight" mode. In many ways, that person has regressed to a more primitive, animalistic state, where he looks for and perceives physical cues rather than more complex, abstract verbal cues; his cortical brain takes a backseat to his limbic brain.[132] Chronically hyper-aroused men lose the ability to interpret their own emotions. The basic function of feelings is to get

---

[130] Leary, Joy Degruy. *Post Traumatic Slave Syndrome: America's Legacy of Enduring Injury and Healing* (Milwaukee: Uptone Press, 2005) Pgs. 114-134.
[131] Ibid. Pgs. 114- 134. Leary
[132] Ibid.

people to pay attention to their environment so that they can take adaptive action. Emotional arousal is part of Nature's design; a reaction to the environment that is designed to stimulate goal-directed action. Instead of seeing the signal of arousal as a sign that it is time to use the cortical brain to figure out how to adapt, the traumatized person/man jumps directly into a fight, flight, or freeze mode. This could well explain why urban homicidal rates are so high. The constant "jacking up" of hyper-arousal reduces one's ability to recognize other emotional signals. [133] Healthy relationships under these circumstances become difficult or impossible, as well as successful performance as a student, employee, or parent. It is not unusual for hyper-vigilant individuals to also resort to avoidance behaviors; effectively shrinking the scope of their lives down to avoid things and people that remind them of the cause of their trauma. I argue that this is one of the many reasons so many African-American men are not with their families; indeed, this assertion is not all-inclusive, however, a prognosis of clinical depression explains why some African-American men are not able to have healthy relationships. It should be taken into account that some African-American men may suffer from undiagnosed clinical depression, and for this reason they are absent from both familial and societal responsibilities.

Secondly, there is dissociation, and under this category there are three subcategories: The first is primary dissociation, the second is secondary dissociation, and third is tertiary dissociation[134]. Primary dissociation describes the split between the sensory and emotional aspects of trauma that can occur during the traumatic event. Instead of perceiving the event as a whole, it is perceived as fragments of sensory information: sight, odors, sounds, and sensations.

[133] Ibid.
[134] Pgs. 114-134. Leary

Afterwards, the person may talk of even "leaving their bodies", or otherwise protecting themselves from pain by observing their trauma as spectators rather than as victims.[135] Ultimately, the breadth of that separation increases and becomes incorporated into the trauma survivor's personality. A split remains, so that some aspects of that person's personality incorporates the pain and fear of their traumatic experience, a reactive measure known among psychologists as tertiary dissociation.[136] When a trauma victim dissociates during the event itself, his chances of developing post-traumatic stress disorder are greater. Dissociation serves the purpose of numbing the impact of the trauma, at the expense of being able to integrate it into one's overall experience, which is the only kind of integration that will heal the wounds that trauma leaves behind.

Dissociative adaptations include a broad range of responses to traumatic experience. Any mental mechanism that disengages a person from what is happening in the external world and tunes one into an internal world is considered a dissociative mechanism. Among them are: daydreaming; fantasizing; the incessant playing of video games; 'watching from outside the body'; going to a "different place"/abusing alcohol or misusing drugs, particularly crack, heroin/ marijuana and malt liquor (for many African-American men); and watching excessive television, particularly music videos where one can fantasize about being wealthy. (Many young African-American men consume these addictive substances and media to give themselves the illusion of being powerful, wealthy, and popular.)[137] In extreme states of dissociation, a person may faint, become catatonic (frozen) or may enter what is known as a "fugue" state.[138] Fugue is defined as an

---

[135] Ibid.
[136] Ibid.
[137] Ibid. Pgs. 114-134. Leary
[138] Ibid.

episode of altered consciousness that causes the individual to wander; he may do so for hours or days, and does not remember it afterwards. A person who is used to dissociating may find that one's pain is numbed, but that they are also cut off from happier feelings. Dissociated people sometimes report feeling numb, dead, or "on auto-pilot."[139] They may even commit violent acts against others or themselves just to feel something. It is this aspect of dissociation in my view that lies at the root of the fecklessness and the culture of anomie for many African-American men. Dissociation could perhaps be as great a social problem as hyper-arousal. Known also as "learned helplessness", some could describe the listlessness of some African-American men on street corners, in front of convenient stores, and around bars an example of dissociation. When an abused person gives up trying, frequent dissociation suggests that they have lost a sense of control over their life and emotions alike, sinking into a state of defeat. This form of helplessness can be associated with unremitting racism in this country.[140] Nevertheless, those who dissociate or give up on life completely are not so likely to commit violence. They are, however, at greater risk of being completely defeated by trauma.[141]

In conclusion, social factors combined with negative mental anguish have created the perfect environment for many African-American men to suffer from clinical depression. The objectives for Chapter 4 are creating a theological perspective for combating social circumstances (and incarceration in particular) and developing a theological hermeneutic for integrating a real meaningful ministry for African-American men who are truly suffering, silently, with clinical depression.

---

[139] Ibid.
[140] Ibid.
[141] Ibid. Leary

# Chapter 4

## A THEOLOGICAL REFLECTION
## FOR AFRICAN-AMERICAN MEN

### Theological Reflections; Theological Interpretations & Applications for Clinical Depression; The Integration of Biblical Interpretation & Praxis; The Demoniac, African-American Men and Community Responses

"No Black Man in America is ever mentally healthy."

*-Anonymous*

"Who really, really gives a damn about the Black Man in America?"

*-Anonymous*

"Now, as then, we find ourselves bound, first without, then within, by the nature of our categorization. And escape is not effected through a bitter railing against this trap; it is as though this very striving were the only motion needed to spring the trap upon us. We take our shape, it is true, within and against that cage of reality bequeathed us at our birth; and yet it is precisely through our dependence on this reality that we are most endlessly betrayed."

*-James Baldwin, Notes of a Native Son*

### Theological Reflections

The story of the demoniac in (Mark 5:1-20; Matt 8:28-34; Luke 8:26-39) shows both the hope in and limitations of disability studies - as applied to theological understanding when it is read as a story of severe mental illness. On the one hand, the demoniac is a man, suffering like so many African-American men today, with a stigmatized mental disease. Although Matthew's account of the story in (Matt. 8:28) asserts that there are two men who are "possessed" with devils, Luke's account agrees with Mark that it is one man (Luke 8:27). That notwithstanding, all three of these narratives agree that the man is experiencing some severe problems. Matthew's account cites that the two men were "...exceedingly fierce, so that no man might pass by the way."[142] Moreover, Luke cites that the man "...ware no clothes, neither abode in any house, but in the tombs."[143] Luke's narrative also mentions that "...he is bound with chains and in fetters." [144] This aspect of Luke's narrative coincides with Mark's narrative on how incarceration was a methodology to control this man, whose mental capacity was problematic.

Furthermore, both Mark and Luke reference the response of the man responding to Jesus by saying his name is Legion (Mark 5:9 and Luke 8:30). Many biblical scholars believe that this reference displays the political oppression or domination of the Roman Empire on oppressed men who are acting as psychopaths to demonstrate their resistance to Roman oppression.[145] In the African-American commentary *True to Our Native Land* Emerson B. Powery, a biblical scholar, argues that "That troublesome quality of black life in slavery was psychologically disturbing. This does not suggest a condition of neurosis; rather the indication is that one's psychological well-being was continually challenged by constant confrontation with the insanity of slavery."[146] Also in the book, another African-American biblical scholar, Stephanie B. Crowder, says, "... he is restored to his

---

[142] Matt. 8:28. KJV Bible
[143] Ibid. Luke 8:27
[144] Ibid Luke 8:2
[145] Blount, Brian. et al. *True to Our Native Land: An African-American Commentary* (Minneapolis: Fortress Press, 2007) Pgs. 130-131.
[146] Ibid. Pgs. 130-131.

right mind and his rightful place in society because he was disrupted and from a destroyed community."[147] On the other hand, while miraculous cures may not be available for those living with mental illnesses, those suffering with clinical depression can indeed be restored from the debilitating effects of it.

The story of the Gerasene demoniac appears in Mark's Gospel, the narrative I use for this context, and we see Jesus within a long teaching section with parables (3:19- 4:34) and may relieve narrative tension with its bizarre, yet entertaining details. More specifically, the story occurs immediately after Jesus calmed the waters and winds of a storm on the Sea of Galilee, which he and his disciples were crossing (4:35- 41). Having just witnessed Jesus' ability to control natural phenomena, the disciples were left a bit shaky-legged, wondering as others in the Gospel already had, "Who then is this?" (4:41). The crossing "to the other side" (4:35; 5:1) is important because it is the first time in the Gospel that Jesus takes his ministry into predominantly Gentile territory, considered ritually unclean, also signaled by the presence of pigs (5:11-13) because Jews were not allowed to eat, let alone keep swine. The narrative emphasizes this point explicitly by describing Jesus' first encounter in the foreign territory as a man with "an unclean spirit", typically referred to as the Gerasene demoniac. In a Gospel that clips along with apocalyptic urgency, the story of this demon possession captures the reader's attention because of its length; twenty verses, the Gerasene demoniac story is the longest healing story in Mark's Gospel. Its relative length invites a sort of settling into its story world.

The plot has three overlapping foci, each of which I will elaborate on and relate to severe mental illness. It describes first the demoniac's situation or experience;

[147] Ibid. Pg. 169.

then the surrounding community's usual response to the demoniac; and ultimately Jesus' exorcism of the demon from the man. From the vantage point of where he had been living among the tombs near the mountains, the demoniac witnessed Jesus' arrival and went to meet him. The demoniac had been living in the tombs for some time, engaging in self-destructive behavior and howling day and night (5:2, 5). Apparently with some success early on, the surrounding community had often restrained the man but was no longer able to do so because he had grown so strong that he was able to break the chains that bound him (5:3-4). However, Jesus proved stronger than the demons, demanding that if they came out of the man he would permit them to enter into a herd of pigs instead, which the demons promptly did and rushed to their destruction over a cliff (5:8-13). Jesus' action made the community afraid, and the man previously possessed by the demon wanted to leave with Jesus, who refused his request and instead commanded him to go home and tell everyone about what had happened to him (5:18-20).

## Theological Interpretation and Application for Clinical Depression

Some scholars may object to interpreting Mark's story of the demoniac in terms of mental illness today because modern, Western notions of "self" that ground contemporary psychology contrast greatly with what has been argued as the concept of self for the ancient 1st century Mediterranean personality. Certainly, examining the 1st century Mediterranean context of the story of the demoniac elicits useful insights that expand and can transform one's understanding of the text. However, the demand to see the text only through this lens at the exclusion or denigration of other perspectives threatens the idea that biblical texts are living traditions that are challenged and renewed by lived experience of ongoing generations of Christians. Given the fact that throughout Western history people believed that behaviors associated with what is referred to as mental illness to be demon possession, the demoniac story of Mark 5 and others like it certainly contributed to the stigmatization and poor treatment of the mentally ill. The mentally ill were perceived as weak-willed or somehow flawed to have given the demon - even Satan himself - a foothold in their lives, perhaps even welcoming evil itself. In addition, what was associated with the demonic or Satan was often perceived to be violent, and so the mentally ill were feared, segregated, restrained, and even executed.[148] Although other theories of mental illness have come to dominate since the 18th century, the theories of a spiritual cause or demonic possession still persist within many cultures and communities today. Thus, many people continue to believe that African-American men who are clinically depressed are "evil" or "cursed" by God. Nonetheless, interpreting the demoniac story of Mark 5:1-19, Matthew 8:28-34 and Luke 8:26-39 as being that of a person with mental illness or a case of severe undiagnosed clinical depression provides an opportunity not only to understand how such texts may contribute to this stigmatization, but also to explore the textual resources for changing those perceptions or reexamining mental illnesses and clinical depression.

Two models within disability studies are useful for interpreting the story of the demoniac of Mark 5. First, the medical model understands disability as a loss of function or ability of a particular body part; that the disability itself lies within the body of the individual and is therefore a medical or biological condition. The goal here is to correct, cure, or restore that loss of function and ability in order to bring the affected area back into "normal" range. Secondly, in contrast, the minority or social group model argues that the problem of disability does not reside with a

---

[148] Toensing, Holly Joan. *Living Among the Tombs: Society, Mental Illness, and Self-Destruction in Mark 5:1-20* (Atlanta: Society of Biblical Literature, 2007)

particular body part of the individual, but in the way society creates physical and attitudinal barriers that limit a person's ability to achieve some measure of success within society. It comes from the perspective that society not only stigmatizes disabled bodies as flawed, inferior, dangerous, and dependent, but also erects social and physical barriers to marginalize, segregate, devalue and discriminate against people with disabilities.

In the context of the biblical story, Jesus confronts a man who is suffering from demon possession, which could be synonymous with clinical depression today. Both the Gerasene demoniac and many African-American men are marginalized, stigmatized, and suffering from alienation in society. Furthermore, the text is explicit in making the reader aware of the man's history of containment or incarceration (5:3-4) which demonstrates the circumstance of this man being perceived as a villain. The self-proclaimed name of the demons, which the man responded back to Jesus, was "legion" (λεγιών in Greek) which was a designation of a military command of Roman soldiers.[149] Some scholars explored the 1st century Mediterranean experience of the Roman military as suggestive of what may have caused the demon possession; in other words, oppression and economic colonization may have been key elements in the man's condition and mental state of being.

Recalling Frantz Fanon's contemporary theory of the "Manichaeism" of colonization, these interpretations highlight the degree to which Roman techniques for military conquests and colonization terrorized populations. In the experience of villagers in Palestine, they argue, the Romans legions "would more than once have attacked their villages unmercifully, burning their houses, slaughtering or

---

[149] Ibid. Pgs. 132-141.

enslaving the people, plundering their goods".[150] The population could do little but comply, while using indirect means of protest - for example, by expressing the hopelessness and madness of their existence through the supposed experience of demon possession. Thus, demon possession was a sanctioned way to act and speak out against one's oppressed situation, a strategy then vicariously participated in by many in the oppressed community.[151] According to this theory, the community begging Jesus to leave after they saw the former demoniac in his right mind (5:17) demonstrates their frustration with Jesus for removing their indirect form of protest against the Roman authority (oppression).[152] This theory rightly highlights how environmental stressors significantly influence the way that people view and respond to the world around them and could contribute to the development of mental illness.[153] Nonetheless, mental illness can strike regardless of social status; it does not afflict just those who are marginalized or oppressed by society. Moreover, such theories suggest mental illness is not just experience; it is a rational reaction, choice, or strategy. Severe mental illness is not experienced as a rational choice or conscious strategy, as if one can turn it on and off.[154]

Regardless of the degree to which environmental stressors cause demon possession, all three Gospels describe how, once inside, the demon-possessed (or clinically depressed) person changes and became unrecognizable as a human being: like a wild animal, the demoniac broke shackles and chains meant to subdue him (5:4) was apparently unclothed (5:15) and continually wandering isolated places howling (5:5). The demon within the man - not the man himself - responded to Jesus' question and commands. (5:7-12). Those who experience severe mental

---

[150] Ibid. Pg. 135.
[151] Ibid.
[152] Ibid.
[153] Ibid.
[154] Ibid. Toensing

illness often describe too that something descends into their bodies and takes control of them, often resulting in uncharacteristic human speech and behavior. Stewart Govig describes the almost animal-like language that regularly emitted from his son John, who was diagnosed with schizophrenia: "he would make urgent, high-pitched, strange subvocal sounds. At times what seemed like a dog's muffled bark broke through the stormy monologue."[155] According to Stewart, these episodes were often accompanied by hyperactive, disorganized activity, which is also associated with some forms of severe mental illness. Once, during an episode of these voices, Stewart Govig's son demanded that his father stop the van he was driving, and the moment it stopped, "the grimacing youth burst out the side door to commence to a rapid, circular, jerky pace."[156] As quoted by Kay Redfield Jamison, a close friend of Drew Sopirak, she poignantly describes similar characteristics of Drew during one of his hospitalizations from a severe form of bipolar disorder:

I remember when [Drew] was hospitalized in D.C. and I went to visit him. His mom left to get dinner, and he laid his head in my lap, curled up in the fetal position. I saw with my eyes the man's face I knew as Drew, but my ears heard another creature. Something else seemed to live in his shell. Someone other than Drew brought words to his lips or created his awkward, disturbing actions. As he rubbed his head, as though to bring his thoughts to some sort of sanity, I looked at him and wondered where my friend had disappeared to. This monster had taken over. He was gaunt and had not shaved in weeks. His skin was sallow and his cheeks sunken; each movement appeared painful. I did not know this person he had become. The more he talked the more my fear for him grew.[157]

Like the demoniac in Mark 5, Drew seemed completely controlled by something else that pulled him further and further away from anything recognizably human;

---

[155] Ibid. Pg. 137.
[156] Ibid.
[157] Ibid. Toensing

verily I say, to one degree or another, this is the same "condition" we find many African-American men in, both historically and presently.

## The Integration of Biblical Interpretation and Praxis

The precipice of death loomed in the life of the demoniac as described in Mark 5. To emphasize its constant presence, the text states three times that the tombs possessed the man's haunt, away from society and community (5:2, 3, 5). In fact, he "had a home" there, perhaps among tombs designed to resemble small houses and temples. However, the Greek verb that was used is in the imperfect form, and expresses the sense that though the man did come habitually to live among the tombs, he had not truly found a home there. Death, though close, has not yet settled.[158] The demoniac continually bruising and cutting himself with stones surely brought him closer to death's door over time (5:5). He literally and spatially occupied the luminal state of being "the living dead" - alive, but for all practical purposes, already dead. Similarly, death can be precariously close at hand for African-American men who suffer mental illness, whether it is bipolar disorder, schizophrenia, or clinical depression. When a man is suffering with clinical depression, his state of being is definitely like "the living dead" as described in the biblical text of Mark 5:1-20, Mark 8:28-34, and in Luke. Thus, as mental illness increases, so too does dramatic increases in successful and unsuccessful suicide attempts and a range of other violent behavior towards one's self and others.

Given the persistence and pervasiveness of mental illness, clinical depression leaves many African-American men mentally tortured and drained. Na'im Akbar, a research psychologist at Florida State University, describes the feelings of African-

---

[158] Ibid.

American men who are suffering from clinical depression as "being frightened of the world; to be walled off from it and harangued by voices; to see life as distorted faces and shapes and colors; to lose constancy and trust in one's brain: for most, the pain is beyond conveying."[159] This description of mental anguish explains the similarities between the Gerasene demoniac and African-American men suffering from clinical depression in urban areas of poverty; both display the isolation from community, either due to one's own withdrawal from society or from the attrition of friends and family, which invariably worsens the situation. Sometimes even if others do succeed at making connections with a clinically depressed person, the nature of the connections can exacerbate the struggle because of the mental and emotional stress that the person is suffering.

## The Demoniac, African-American Men, and Community Response

The relevant question for a transformative church is: How does the community (congregation) deal with the demoniacs within our midst (many African-American men) in today's society? We know that the biblical text says "No one could restrain him" (5:3); this action is then intensified in the text by its developed description of means, frequency, and intent of that restraint: "not even with a chain; for he had often been restrained with shackles and chains...to subdue him" (5:3b-4).[160] For this community, restraining the demoniac may not have only kept the man from the place of death -the tombs - but also possibly from death itself. The tombs were places for the dead; places where demons, rejects, incorrigibles and irredeemable people were believed to lurk. Hellenistic culture allowed regular visits to the tombs of a loved one as an acceptable funerary practice, while self-

---

[159] Akbar, Na'im. *Breaking the Chains of Psychological Slavery* (Tallahassee: Mind Productions & Associates, 1996) Pgs. 14-26.
[160] The Holy Bible.

mutilation, including tattooing, was associated with pagan funerary rites (Lev. 19:28; 21:5; Deut. 14:1).[161] However, because the demoniac was doing these things "always night and day" (5:5) community members may have begun to worry about the outcome of his self-destructive action. Thus, it is conceivable that they would have used restraints to keep this man from taking his own life. Alternatively, the community may have repeatedly attempted to restrain the possessed man to end his nuisance. While graveyards were typically in isolated areas away from the boundaries of a community, the shrieking of the demoniac may have echoed across the land, preventing the community from forgetting about the man's presence. His noises may have been a public nuisance that restraint could temper. Similarly, the restraints may have also represented insurance of community protection from the man. The text details the extent to which the man was apparently self-destructive; was it just a matter of time before he would lash out at others? Had he, indeed, already done so? While the text suggests that the demoniac kept to the tombs and mountains, the Greek verb "δέω", meaning "to restrain or bind" was often associated with imprisonment (5:3-4).[162] Were the villagers in a violent rage so great that they wanted to remove that possibility altogether and to control or limit his rage? After all, the Greek word "δαμάσαι" means "to subdue" which suggests taming the unpredictability of a wild animal in order to gain control of it and then to manipulate its behavior.[163] Bound and gagged, the demoniac could pose no danger to the community and he could be punished for any past crimes or simply removed from society.

Institutionalization, which is the process of putting people into prisons, correctional facilities or mental institutions, is often the way The United States has

---

[161] Ibid. Toensing. Pg. 138.
[162] Ibid. Pgs. 138-141.
[163] Ibid.

dealt with many African-American men who are suffering from clinical depression. Institutionalization, criminalization, and incarceration in the U.S. have gone toward creating the largest prison system in the world - the Prison Industrial Complex. Under such conditions, the fate of African-American men is devoid of dignity, healing, and wholeness. Being confined to a jail cell and promulgated as a miscreant is not dissimilar to the experience of the Gerasene demoniac who was restrained time and time again (Mark 5:4). This is the usual pattern for those with mental illness; it is a revolving door of re-institutionalization in jails and prisons across the country, with no palpable end in sight in either affective policy or practice. For many African-American men, "chains and shackles" have physically shape-shifted into prison cells, and worst of all, have metaphysically shifted into lifelong criminalization, alienation, and all too often social and economic oblivion. The text makes an assertion in Mark (5:3) that the attempt was made to incarcerate the man; perhaps the most exhausted form of institutionalization used to control the demoniac African-American man is incarceration. Incarceration is a very important aspect of what is ravaging the African-American community because so many African-American men are imprisoned. The Church must articulate its vision and voice of justice to combat the disproportionate incarceration of African-American men being bound, "δέω", just like the Gerasene demoniac, through the federal, state, and county correctional systems.

Valid questions aimed at unearthing a truth-based dialogue about mental health among African-American men include: How would it feel, living in the richest country in the world, earning less than $10,000 a year, while watching people on television live lavishly? What is it like for African-American men who are living in housing projects, not gainfully employed, while simultaneously watching videos of people living in mansions? Indeed, questions like these and their responses highlight the trauma, the reality; a significant factor of depression for many African-American men. Unfortunately, this is how many inner city African-American men experience life daily. African-Americans are approximately 13% of this nation's population but are disproportionally incarcerated; over 1 million African-American men are currently in prison and another 3.5 million are on parole or probation or have felony records, having neither voting rights or good jobs, limited earning potential, and are enduring severe family and community consequences because of it.[164] Therefore, the stifling power and the controlling affects on the whole of the African-American community is staggering.[165] For every 100,000 Americans, 730 are incarcerated, and this only includes federal and state prisons.[166] These numbers do not include local jails and people under probation. Furthermore, when you dissect the 730; for every 100,000 white males in America approximately 461 of them are incarcerated, but for every 100,000 African-American males the figure leaps to 3,250.[167]

To contextualize the severity of the problem, it is helpful to place this African-American incarceration pandemic within a larger context. In 1993, the last year of legal apartheid in South Africa, there were 581 black inmates per 100,000 black South Africans.[168] In America, we have almost four times that number and, supposedly, we are not living under apartheid.[169] Could there be a correlation between depression and this country's incarceration rate? How are the cumulative effects of African-American men and the dynamics of oppression, distress, and racism promoting this alarming incarceration of African-American men? When did

---

[164] Boothe, Demico. *Why Are So Many Black Men In Prison?* (Memphis, TN: Full Surface Publishing, 2007) Pg. 61.
[165] Ibid.
[166] Kunjufu, Jawanza. *State of Emergency: Why We Must Save African-American Males.* (Chicago: African-American Images, 2001) Pgs. 109-144.
[167] Ibid.
[168] Ibid.
[169] Ibid.

this high incarceration start and what is the cause of it? Moreover, what perpetuates this pandemic and how is depression connected to it? These are more of the valid and vital questions that The Church must observe and engage to bring about transformation for African-American men.

For one, the so-called "War on Drugs" is in actuality a war on poor, clinically depressed African-American men. Between 1980 and 1993, Presidents Ronald Reagan and George Bush Sr. cut federal spending on employment and training by nearly 50% while corrections spending increased by 521%. Federal, state, and local funding of justice systems literally exploded in the two decades leading up to the year 2000. On average, direct federal, state, and local expenditures for police grew by 16%, court costs grew by 58%, prosecution and legal services by 152%, public defense by 259%, and corrections by 668%, while county spending increased by 711% and state spending surged by 848%. In California, the ratio is eight inmates to every one college student. (California allocates $31,000 to lock up a youth in a juvenile detention center, but less than $6,000 to teach elementary and high school students.)[170] Concurrently, the backlashes of this along with not having available mass opportunities for meaningful and gainful employment in most sectors of black society worked correspondently with racism, miseducation, and drug proliferation to destroy African-American communities.

Subsequently, the aggregate effect of the abandonment of urban areas started the explosion of high crime in inner cities; unquestionably the crime, coupled with the misuse of the law, created absolute mayhem in most inner cities. Ironically, it is during this period that the government characterized its "war" tactics to eradicate drugs as "The War on Drugs" and "The War on Crime" when effectually speaking

---

[170] Ibid.

it is a "War on Those Who Do Crime", particularly vulnerable unemployed black and brown males. This charge is not merely my personal opinion; the same has long been touted by a few activists and legislators who are concerned about the record numbers of African-Americans being jailed for outrageously long periods of time for non-violent drug offenses. "The rapid expansion of the U.S. Prison Industrial Complex has been fueled by the so-called War on Drugs", said Rep. Maxine Waters (D-California).[171] She has cited findings from a Human Rights Watch report showing African-American men are imprisoned for drug crimes at thirteen times the rate of white men even though black and white drug users rates are similar, and that in sheer numbers there are far more white American drug users than black users overall. A recent study done by the Justice Department shows that half of those charged in federal courts for drugs offenses had no prior convictions and a significant number had no prior arrest. It also acknowledges that less than 1% of those jailed and given stiff mandatory sentences by the federal courts fit the profile of drug kingpins. Thus one could argue that African-American males in large part are, at most, pawns of an ineffective judicial system and vulnerable to what Jewelle Taylor Gibbs describes in *Young Black and Male in America:* "...living unequivocally unenviable lives of almost total rejection."[172]

To get more specific, the implementation of the mandatory minimum guidelines and the "Crack vs. Power" law are the major causative factors behind the rate of increase of federal prisons more than doubling the rate of increase of state prisons in the passing years. These laws set the slate for the focus and efforts of federal as well as state law enforcement agencies nationwide to aim at targeting young black men in the ghettos of urban America and making them the scapegoats of America's

---

[171] Boothe, Demico. *Why Are So Many Black Men In Prison?* (Memphis: Full Surface Publishing, 2007) Pgs. 79-92.
[172] Gibbs, Jewelle. et al. *Young Black and Male in America: An Endangered Species.* (Dover, Massachusetts: Auburn House Publishing Company) Pgs. 1-5.

new "War on Drugs" and "War on Crime." The strict drug laws introduced in New York in 1973 by then Governor Nelson Rockefeller inspired the sentiment behind the configuration of these harsh draconian laws. Under the "Rockefeller Drug Laws", possession of four ounces of narcotics carries a mandatory fifteen to life sentence. As a result of who was targeted by the New York law enforcement, 94% of the more than 20,000 people that were subsequently sentenced on drug felonies in New York State shortly after the law was implemented were black and Latino, although, as I've said, the U.S. government's figures show that blacks and Latinos do not use illicit drugs at a greater rate than whites.[173] Far too many African-American men are being prosecuted at the federal level for drug possession and the sale of crack cocaine despite documented racial disparities. As recently as 2003, former Attorney General John Ashcroft publicly sent a memo out to all federal prosecutors ordering them to step up and seek to give out the highest sentences possible.[174] (It should be noted that in the State of New York and in some other states as well, the draconian Rockefeller Drug Laws and other laws of the type are currently being either reconstructed or considered for repeal supposedly due to the many men, especially African-American men, who are/were unfairly disenfranchised by them.)

Almost entire generations of African-American men have already been criminalized because of illegal drugs, to the point that we have significantly more young black men in prison than in college. So much so that some people now refer to prisons in America as "The Black Man's University."[175] Currently there are over 1 million African-American men in prison and just 600,000 in higher education. In Indiana in 2001, black men comprised 4% of the state's population and 40% of

---

[173] Ibid. Boothe
[174] Ibid.
[175] Ibid.

them were in prison. Of the other 60%, less than one-third of them were in college or any form of higher education. Using the state of Michigan as an example, in the year 2000 there were 24,300 blacks, most of whom were men, in the state of Michigan's prisons and 21,454 blacks, most of whom were females, in the state's colleges and universities.[176] There is a direct linkage between this fact and the fact that between 1985 and 2000 Michigan increased corrections spending by 1.11 billion dollars, or 227%. It costs the state of Michigan $28,000 a year to incarcerate a person, which is the equivalent of what it could cost the state to pay the annual tuition of five students at one of its public universities. Instead, like many state legislatures, Michigan's political leaders have implicitly committed to a preference for paying for an African-American male to go to prison rather than supporting the financial burden of their college attendance.[177] Therefore, our crime problems and the question of punishment for crimes cannot really be properly analyzed and understood apart from the larger social, political, and economic context from which they emerge. Black crime and the position of black men within the nation's system of criminal justice administration are unswervingly related to past *and* present social disadvantages; therefore, those disadvantages can best be understood through the consideration of black men's overall social status and mental state of being.

Consequently, one must consider that too many African-Americans were raised in poverty and continue certain relevant traditions into adulthood, setting the stage for them to develop an inclination toward considering criminal activity as a way of life and as a means to an end, and especially so with the men and boys. The social position of a group of people has definitive links to that group's economic

---

[176] Ibid.

[177] Kitwana, Bakari. *Young Blacks and the Crisis in African-American Culture: The Hip Hop Generation* (New York: Perseus Books Group, 2002) Pgs. 3-24.

situation, and the groups itself does not solely determine its position. Much of the racial differences apparent in who commits certain crimes have direct ties to income levels and class differences and those extreme concentrations of poverty in our inner city neighborhoods lead to higher levels of crime and violence being perpetrated by the inhabitants of those areas, which in turn creates the "need" for more and different types of policing in those areas that are obviously not designed to "protect and serve" in the most humane and sensitive fashion. To the contrary, Christian Parenti, in his enlightening work *Lockdown America: Police and Prisons in the Age of Crisis* argues that this is part of a 1980's/90's nationwide trend in policing designed to put a certain "force" back into the police industry:

For centuries, "urban" has been synonymous with filth, lawlessness, and danger, but in recent years cities have also taken on a renewed economic and cultural importance as sites of accumulation, speculation, and innovation profit making. For cities to work as such, they must be, or at last appear and feel safe. If the economic restructuring of the eighties and nineties intensified urban poverty, it also created new, gilded spaces that are increasingly *threatened by poverty*. This polarization of urban space and social relations has in turn required a new layer of regulation and exclusion, so as to protect the new hyper-aestheticized, playground quarters of the postmodern from their flipsides of misery. This contradiction, between the danger of cities and their value, has spawned yet another revolution in American law enforcement: the rise of zero tolerance/quality of life policing.[178]

This seemingly "open season" on African-American men and teenagers by policing forces is a pattern that too often has repeated itself throughout the 1980's and 1990's. The mass demonstrations, including those that followed the Rodney King beating in Los Angeles, Malice Green's murder in Detroit, Johnny Gammage's murder in Pittsburgh, Abner Louima's beating in New York City, and

---

[178] Parenti, Christian. *Lockdown America: Police and Prisons in the Age of Crisis* (Verso, 2000)

# A THEOLOGICAL REFLECTION FOR AFRICAN-AMERICAN MEN

Amadou Diallo's murder by officers in New York City reflect overwhelming frustration and growing cynicism about policing that has reached an all-time high. The collapse of trust in law enforcement and the vilification of black men through crime legislation certainly play an important role in the views that black men share about legislation, law enforcement, and criminal justice.

Concomitantly, big industrial companies began to move overseas in large numbers in order to take advantage of cheap labor, leaving minorities in the inner cities jobless. This caused many family breakups, therefore many of the women ended up on welfare while many of the men became hopeless and started to indulge in drug dealing, engage in substance abuse, and other criminal activities to make money. (Note - In two famous cases of African-American men residing in inner cities during the Reagan-Bush era -Rodney King in Los Angeles and Malice Green of Detroit - both men had experienced job lost and social displacement. Thus they experienced the punitive difficulties of being estranged from their wives and children and struggled with illegal drug addictions and had various bouts with the law. I would like to suggest that these particular men were suffering from undiagnosed clinical depression. This is a perfect example of what happens to many inner city African-American men vulnerable to the economy, and displaced in community. They become victims of a racist judicial system; they lack emotional support and nurturance, and they are not connected to a viable church that can minister effectively to African-American men.) These same symptoms of depression are apparent in so many African-American men, particularly in inner city America. Despite these obvious examples of clinical depression, it is disheartening that the predominant American culture continues to treat African-American men as outcasts, villains, and felonious criminals rather than recognize the need for an objective prognosis for African-American men.

Louis Uchitelle, a journalist covering economics for the New York Times, in his book *The Disposable American* poignantly described in a chapter entitled *The Consequences – Undoing Sanity* the cataloging of damage that results from layoffs and incapacitating emotional illness that almost never appears on the lists that economists, politicians, sociologists, union leaders, business school professors, management consultants, and journalists compile. He further argues, "There is much discussion of income loss, downward mobility, a decrease in family cohesion, a rise in the divorce rate, the unwinding of communities, and the impact on children."[179] One can adduce that the given factors should be studied psychoanalytically for how they impact black folk and cause black people, black families, and black communities to suffer from clinical depression. It is preposterous that all of this information is well documented for European Americans, who are in many cases, middle class in our society, while no serious researchers have produced sanitized and humanizing descriptions of the anguish and animosity felt by many African-American men who are often poor and have gone protracted periods without gainful employment. Louis Uchitelle cites in his book a psychoanalyst, Dr. Theodore Jacobs, who says, "There are many people who do not want to face that trauma again and to some degree they lose a sense of reality."[180] Perhaps this statement describes the anomie and lack of initiative that many African-American men feel concerning looking for employment.

Clinical depression perpetuates a feeling of worthlessness. It also causes a deep level of frustration, which is expressed in a number of ways but primarily through homicide and suicide. Does this explain why African-American men kill African-American men disproportionally in many urban cities in the United States? If

---

[179] Uchitelle, Louis. *The Disposable American: Layoffs and Their Consequences* (New York: Vintage Books, 2007) Pgs. 178-191.
[180] Ibid.

African-American males are such good killers, why don't they kill everybody and anybody? One possible cogent explanation could be that people who feel they are without a future have the propensity to become dangerous primarily *to one another*. This is one point that must be raised when ministering to African-American men. It is arguably delusional to suggest that men who are under such anguish and affliction could do anything but be bilious and crestfallen to one another. Many believe the African-American community is in a serious state of emergency and actually is experiencing a "silent genocide".[181] Terrie M. William's argues in her book that the severity of depression in the African-American community is extraordinarily high.[182] Moreover, she is alarmed that we are not even talking about it in our community, nor our churches and places of worship; rather we are misdiagnosing the malady as "going nuts", "being crazy", and describes the situation of African-American men particularly as "living totally out of control" and "evil".[183] Furthermore, as aforementioned, we are witnessing suicide on the rise in the African-American community. Twenty-five per 100,000 African-American men are victims of suicide.[184] What will it take for us to begin to do something to help African-American men experiencing this level of crisis? This question ought to be raised in every faith community, especially those congregations that are ministering in communities where African-American men reside, work, and languish.

Bakari Kitwana perfectly illuminates the subject in his book *The Hip Hop Generation* where he trenchantly describes the abomination, astringency, and desertion felt by African-American men who have over time adopted a callous

---

[181] Williams, Terrie M. *Black Pain: It Just Looks Like We're Not Hurting* (New York: Scriber, 2008) Pg. 1-30.
[182] Ibid.
[183] Ibid.
[184] U.S. Statistical Abstract, 2000

attitude and emotional state due to social pressures. Evidenced among my surveyed focus group from Kaighn Avenue Baptist Church is one young man who while talking on the subject of how African-American men feel emotionally, described the attitude of many African-American men as being "pissed off" or "mad as hell" due to "the constant stress and strain of prejudice, racism, and economic inequities in this country"[185] - Kitwana vividly illustrates and defines this same emotional description of African-American men in a chapter in his book entitled *Young, Don't Give a Fuck and Black*. And thus, the persona of African-American men is often promulgated as ferocious, cruel, barbarous and criminally maniacal. Regrettable, this derogatory caricature is fully accepted by many African-American men as their persona and demeanor and this caricature is exploited, marketed and advertised to the entire world. Kitwana further argues that African-American men are thus mislabeled in blanket fashion in society as "gun toting, ruthless, violent, criminal, and cold-hearted killers."[186] When in all actuality these men are probably crying out for help from mental anguish and social alienation: clinical depression. This is a travesty; unfortunately no one appears to be reading the symptoms of obvious mental illness in many of our men.

In conclusion, suffice it to say, there is a need for a transformative vision for African-American men, particularly those men who are suffering from clinical depression. In addition, there is a tremendous need for insightful scriptural perspectives on the issue that will attract, involve, and minister to clinically depressed black men efficiently and effectively. This humanistic task fall squarely onto the shoulders of The Church; The Church must engage new and innovative

---

[185] Braswell, William. A mailman in Cherry Hill, New Jersey. Interviewed by author, 25th of July 2008.
[186] Kitwana, Bakari. *The Hip Hop Generation: Young Blacks and the Crisis in African-American Culture* (New York: Perseus Books, 2002) Pgs. 121-141.

A THEOLOGICAL REFLECTION FOR AFRICAN-AMERICAN MEN

directives to educate, equip, and minister to African-American men, and must begin doing so expeditiously.

# Chapter 5

## DEVELOPING A MODEL FOR LIBERATION & TRANSFORMATION

### Theological Solutions for African-American Men

### The Survey; The Method; Meaning in Life Questionnaire; Moving Towards a Theology of Wholeness for African-American Men

There can be no vulnerability without risk;
and there can be no community without vulnerability;
and there can be no peace - ultimately no life - without community.

*M. Scott Peck*

In this chapter, African-American male congregates of Kaighn Avenue Baptist Church completed a survey examining their own personal probability of being clinical depressed. From the results of the survey, it's more than obvious that ministering on the issue of depression is a must. Also, the importance of creating and promoting community engagements and discussions such as this for African-American men as a relevant and visible component of the faith community (The Church) cannot be understated and is vital in creating a network of significant relationships that are characterized by a viable, relevant theology. Working toward that end, the method used in this particular project includes one survey, three Bible studies, a profile of project participants, a summary of surveys and participants, and details of the procedures used.

## The Survey

The purpose of this study was to examine the general emotion of African-American men who worship at Kaighn Avenue Baptist on a regular basis. Due to cultural nuisances within the African-American community and with African-American men in particular, the test was done with promised anonymity for those who participated in the surveys. The survey that I mainly tapped is utilized and heavily promoted by Ed Diener, professor of psychology at the University of Illinois at Urbana-Champaign, and is called *The Meaning in Life Questionnaire,* which was first developed by M.F. Steger, P. Frazier, & S. Oishi. The survey was strictly on a voluntary basis and most participants did not find it tedious to complete them. The survey asked each participate to check the appropriate response anonymously in order to encourage better participation and truthfulness in their responses. There are ten poignant questions in the survey designed to detect undiagnosed clinical depression. The questions are taken from The Network of Depression Centers (NNDC) which is a group of sixteen university Psychiatry and Behavioral Health Department(s) that have come together on depression. The primary goal of the NNDC is to transform and accelerate the understanding and treatment of depressive and bipolar disorders by developing an integrated network of leading depression centers, one of which is the University of Pennsylvania.

## The Method

### Samples and Field Procedures

Contingent data is derived from the University of Pennsylvania's Depression Center, part of the University of Pennsylvania's Department of Psychiatry, which is based on a stratified and multistage area probability sample of persons aged 15 to 54 years old in non-institutional civilian population in the forty-eight contiguous states. In my survey, I used a meld of the questions from the University of Pennsylvania's Behavioral Science Department's Depression Center's Satisfaction along with questions from Life Scale (a measure of an individual's quality of life). Specific information concerning the participants, their lives, existence, and their feelings as significant to their emotional well-being is the basis of the sample. Each question for my Meaning in Life Questionnaire could be answered with the following responses: **1)** absolutely untrue, **2)** mostly untrue, **3)** somewhat untrue, **4)** cannot say true or false, **5)** somewhat true, **6)** mostly true, **7)** absolutely true.

## *Meaning in Life Questionnaire*

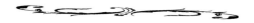

1. I understand my life's meaning.
2. I am looking for something that makes my life feel meaningful.
3. I am always looking for my life's purpose.
4. My life has a clear sense of purpose.
5. I have a good sense of what makes my life meaningful.
6. I have a discovered a satisfying life purpose.
7. I am always searching for something that makes my life feel significant.
8. I am seeking a purpose or mission for my life.
9. My life has no clear purpose.
10. I am searching for meaning in my life.

\* **The men's answers can be found in Appendix C**

The specific purpose of the questionnaire was to examine the feelings of a wide array of men who worship at Kaighn Avenue Baptist and to get a sense of their general mentality about themselves and how they see themselves in terms of earning and life's purpose. Thus, the research was also to give empirical evidence of the argument that was made in Chapter 2. Therefore, in the survey I wanted to get very decisive information on *life's meaning* from these men, believing this survey would have implications of undiagnosed clinical depression within many of my African-American male congregates.

{Note: The survey was taken on Sunday, December 28, 2008 during Sunday school, in order to construct an audience where a diverse group of men are more likely to participate in it. I also wanted to have an opportunity to engage in conversation on the topic of clinical depression so that the participants would be more lucid and comfortable on the subject and have a greater propensity to engage the questions on the survey honestly without being ashamed. Additionally, I wanted to use the holiday season as fulcrum to test my argument on clinical depression, since the holiday season is usually an emotional time and one where suicides typically increase. Before coming to the class with the survey, I arrived unannounced to avoid creating anxiety amongst the men in the class. A total of twenty-five respondents participated in the survey; twenty-two totally completed the survey. For the purposes of this study, the sample was limited to African-American men who live in Camden or the first tier suburbs outside the city; Lindenwold, Sicklerville, and Pennsauken, New Jersey. Those who reside in these areas are either in federally subsidized public housing apartment complexes or prone to be residing in some form of shared housing arrangement with non-familial adults. This criterion resulted in having eighteen valid surveys, which were all completely filled out. Given that this was a men's Sunday school class, everyone in the class was over eighteen years of age. The age of the men in the class ranged from 35-60 years old.}

## Moving Toward a Theology of Wholeness for African-American Men

Theology is indispensable in shaping faith and culture processes. Theologian J. Deotis Roberts speaks forthrightly:

It is just not true that activism is sufficient in itself. The black church needs a theology both for its self-understanding and for its sense of mission. We need to know not merely that we should act; we need to know why we should act. Theology and ministry are inseparable. [187]

Along these lines, theologian Dr. C. Eric Lincoln concludes:

The black church has traditionally relied upon a preached theology...now that era may past. The blacks of this generation, and possibly for generations to come are going to write their own theology in the light of their circumstances and their needs. A white Jesus, whether preached, taught or implied by cultural habits, simply won't do. In a society like ours, he can't do anything for black folks! A white church that is painfully adjunctive to institutional racism - the consequences of which are devastating the whole society - can't do anything for black people. It can't do anything for itself.[188]

The results of the study sustain my hypothesis; by merely reviewing the responses to questions one, three, five, seven, and nine, a conclusion can be reached that the men in the study are befuddled about life's meaning. In question one, the overwhelming response was four, *can't say true or false*, and one, *absolutely untrue*, which indicates frustration concerning one's meaning in life. In question three, the overwhelming response is number four, *can't say true or false*, and two,

---

[187] Roberts, J. Deotis. *The Roots of a Black Future: Family and Church* (Philadelphia, PA: Westminster Press, 1980) Pg. 111.
[188] Lincoln, C. Eric. *Black Church: Christianity and Crisis*, vol. 30, No. 18 (1970) Pg. 226.

*mostly untrue.* In question five, the response was *mostly untrue* and *somewhat true.* In question seven, the response was *can't say true or false*, and *absolutely true.* Finally, in question nine the response was overwhelmingly *absolutely true*, *mostly true*, and the third response was *can't say true or false.* I adduce that the evidence produced by these men participating in this anonymous survey represent both the trauma and dissociative adaptations described in Chapters 2 and 3. The evidence of this survey indicates that some of these men could suffer from at least being unsure of themselves and may be possibly suffering from undiagnosed clinical depression. Significantly, many questions were answered with the response *can't say true or false,* which indicates that many of these men have lost control of their feelings; thereby, many African-American men possibly have moved mentally and emotionally into that stage of dissociation. Thus, the results of the survey are another very strong indication that the urban church must develop a theology that engages and restores vitality to African-American men who are victims of a hegemonic society. In practice, this theology must speak directly to the depressed condition of African-American men.

Upon revisiting these men's survey responses, two salient factors surface. First, responses of emptiness and worthlessness dominated their responses to questions five, nine, and ten. Monitoring the survey takers, I perceived a sense of restlessness and pessimism in the survey results for over half the responses of the men who were surveyed. Next, the answers in questions one, three, five and eight seem to identify with the description of dissociative behaviors of numbness and being "on auto pilot" or insensitive to one's own emotions, and particularly when reviewing the answers to question number four. Where the answer to question four is *can't say true or false,* this response is specifically indicative of clinical depression dissociation; "learned helplessness" or listlessness, which can be described as the behavior often exhibited by many African-American men in urban ghettos loitering without purpose in front of neighborhood stores and on street corners. These dissociative behaviors do suggest helplessness, a loss of control, and emotional and possibly psychological defeat. Very few churches are equipped theologically to engage this kind of clinical depression that the survey suggests exists within many African-American men who, albeit at a minimum, are already attending church. So then what implication does this survey have about those African-American men who are not attending church and not getting any ecclesiastical "food" whatsoever?

So then how does the typical church pursue this prevalent issue within its own African-American male demographic? What theological hermeneutic is necessary to practice a theological construct that empowers the congregation to become a vital tool in the amelioration of African-American men? James H. Evans, Jr., Professor of Systematic Theology at Colgate Rochester Crozer Divinity School, argues in his book *We Shall All Be Changed* that:

One may ask whether African-American theology lacks a social theory upon which to base its analysis of the problems of human society. Or one may ask whether African-American theology is attentive to church organization. Both of these important questions point to an even larger, more comprehensive one: How is African-American theology related to the sociopolitical problems of the world's poor and oppressed? [189]

Professor Evans further argues that African-American practical theology should center on the issues of social/cultural analysis.[190] Therefore, The Church has to acquire new tools to critically and analytically see African-American men as both human and important to its mission of spreading Christianity throughout the world.

---

[189] Evans, James H., Jr. *We Shall All Be Changed* (Minneapolis: Fortress Press, 1997) Pg. 3.
[190] Ibid. Pg. 3.

This methodology Evans suggests must combine a cultural and economic analysis to understanding the oppression of African-American men in particular and the poor in general, in the world.[191] The justification for this assertion is that neither cultural nor economic analysis is biblical or traditional. The content of practical theology is a particular social problem. This content energizes the theological task, while this aspect of theological reflection is most likely to be seen as relevant to the life of the ordinary Christian.[192] In the context of clinical depression within African-American men, The Church must apply practical theology to working towards an applicable hermeneutic of Scripture for African-American men. When this approach is taken, the solutions for ministering to African-American men will be much easier to attain.

The Church must rigorously assume the task of being an instrument of healing for African-American men. The Church must be a transformative agent in society, whereby leading the culture to embrace, encourage, and exhort African-American men. All churches must first examine the moral implications of Christian witness in the world. This witness itself involves three moral movements. According to James H. Evans Jr., first, Christians must engage in moral discernment by examining the hidden desires and fears of people, institutions, and social systems in order to find the sources of impediments to justice and truth. Second, this moral discernment must be guided by moral norms; that is, one must have a set of criteria by which one can determine whether the present social order is just. Thirdly, the rules for Christian living should compel the believer to choose life, freedom and integrity, and move the believer to right action.[193] The aim of The Church is not

---

[191] Ibid.
[192] Ibid. Evans
[193] Ibid. Pg. 4.

simply to preach and have "church" (engage in ritualistic religious practices that do not necessarily require more of a parishioner than passive listening skills). Instead, The Church should lead in transforming the society for justice and righteousness. In the context of clinical depression within African-American men, The Church must clearly engage social issues, economic, and political issues that are the causes of the trauma for many African-American men.

As a sociologist, W.E.B. Du Bois clearly understood the social problems that faced "The Negro" in the late 19th and early 20th centuries when he wrote expressing the experience of being a Negro in America as a dilemma that perhaps best describes the mental and emotional state of many African-American men today in an introspective passage in *The Souls of Black Folk*. Du Bois probes the issue of mental anguish:

Between me and the other world there is ever an unasked question: unasked by some through feelings of delicacy by others through the difficulty of rightly framing it. All, nevertheless, flutter round it. They approach me in a half-hesitant sort of way, eye me curiously or compassionately, and then, instead of saying directly, how does it feel to be a problem? ...At these I smile, or am interested, or reduce the boiling to a simmer, as a problem? I seldom answer a word. And yet, being a problem is a strange experience, - peculiar even for one who has never been anything else, save perhaps in babyhood and in Europe.[194]

I believe that Du Bois expresses the piercing feeling of being constantly traumatized by an unremitting social, racial, economic, and political system. Is this not the promulgation of negative epitaphs that are often depicted by mainstream media where African-American men are characterized as ferocious maniacs and inveterate criminals? What can The Church do to engage this kind of malaise that

---

[194] Du Bois, W.E.B. *The Souls of Black Folk* {New York: Penguin Books, 2003 (1903)} Pg. 54.

has so gripped the African-American man? In the African-American community, the mass devastation is a derivative of our failure to answer this question. Failure to answer this question has wreaked havoc upon most urban areas throughout the United States. The problem with most orthodox American Christian theology is that it does not take seriously the need to deal with this question of African-American men. In too many cases it is American Christian praxis and theology that has created this travesty in the first place, due to America's racist and economic exploitation of people of color historically.

Generally speaking, orthodox American Christian theology does not take seriously the need to deal with this question. Our view of God is the very foundation of what we are, think and do. It influences every single institution in our society. This has serious implications on philosophical, educational, political, economic, and ecclesiastical understandings. Therefore, it is liberating, when done correctly, for both the oppressed and the oppressor to reexamine God's concepts. James Cone says:

The lives of a black slave and white slaveholder were radically different. It follows that their thoughts about divine things would also be different, even though they might sometimes use the same words about God. The life of the slaveholders and others of the culture was that of extending white inhumanity to excruciating limits, involving the enslavement of Africans and the annihilation of Indians. The life of the slave was the slave ship, the auction block, and the plantation regime. It involved the attempt to define himself without the ordinary historical possibilities of self-affirmation. Therefore, when the master and slave spoke of God, they could not possibly be referring to the same reality.[195]

The Church will never really be able to benefit African-American men without reexamining its biblical interpretations and rectifying its God concept, which in

---

[195] Cone, James H. *God of the Oppressed* (New York: Seabury Press, 1975) Pg. 10.

America justifies Manifest Destiny - which is hegemonic and vastly destructive in nature and in practice, particularly to dispossessed people. If The Church wants to minister effectively to African-American men who are dispossessed, wounded, and traumatized by social and economic factors, The Church must create and engage African-American men with a Scripture based theology. Many African-American men do not identify with the God of American Christian theology, a hegemonic God that only identifies with the oppressor and the powerful. African-American men cannot nor will not love a God who does not love them. Consequently, their rejection of Christianity and in many cases, acceptance of Islam is based on a fallacious God concept. The God many African-American men reject is the God of racism, imperialism, materialism, militarism, and every other ideology that negates and neglects African-American men's dignity. In other words, they feel that American Christian religion is never on the side of the disenfranchised and disinherited; many African-American men see Christ on the side of the majority, the powerful, whoever has the might, whoever has the biggest guns and military power.

From a psycho-theological perspective, the problem among African-American men stems from the fact that many are torn between allegiance to a God who wills their destruction and the God who wills their well-being. Those with an unhealthy view of God are typically not wholly interested in the very subject of God or are often engaged in other kinds of self-destructing theologies. However, those who will embrace the God of Scripture can experience triumph in the midst of oppression while their ecclesiastical leaders construct viable theologies via James H. Cone, James H. Evans, Jr., Dwight Hopkins, Anthony Pinn, J. Deotis Roberts and other theologians who are interpreting and reexamining biblical text from new perspectives that speak to African-American men's liberation. (Included within this list are the voices of women, particularly African-American scholars who are womanist theologians and biblical scholars. These women include women like Gay L. Byron, Raquel A. St. Clair, Renita Weems, Katie G. Cannon, and Clarice J. Martin.) The task for The Church in the community is not popularity and large opulent edifices; but to present an unpopular Christ to an oppressed people as the way of salvation. The Church must proclaim a Christ of humiliation and exaltation, abandoning neither. In preaching Jesus, we must make it clear that he is not the Western Christ or the Jesus of chronic suffering, which often precipitates unnecessary and unalleviated pain that is exhibited by many African-American religious theologies. He is the Universal, or the Cosmic Christ. Notwithstanding, at the level of particularity, he identifies with all who are oppressed, marginalized, and abused irrespective of pigmentation, race, class, and gender. The Church must proclaim unequivocally that God (Yahweh) was incarnated in one called Jesus of Nazareth. The Logos became flesh in one who would be considered a failure.[196] This within itself makes Jesus an outcast in America, because America loves a winner. Nonetheless, when Jesus was born, Rome ruled the then known world including Jesus' native Palestine. In other words, Jesus' country was a subject nation. He knows what it means to be: a slave, a minority, poor, locked out, homeless, persecuted and incarcerated. This is an extremely critical psychological breakthrough; this biblical perspective of Jesus Christ being able to identify with constant humiliation and oppression immediately makes the message of Christ germane to African-American men traumatized by American ethos. Yet, Christ in the midst of this vicious oppression and humiliation is victorious - and both physically and spiritually whole. Christ in his humiliation looks like what African-American men are. In his exaltation, he looks like what African-American men shall become.

---

[196] St. John 1:14. KJV Bible.

Now, it is an understatement to say that many African-Americans hate themselves (one of the malicious side effects of American Christian theology and racism). This is a crucial point to be observed by The Church because anyone who hates himself or herself cannot be rightly related to God. Columbus Salley and Ronald Behm, in their important book *What Color is Your God* said:

The negative forces in operation during the period of slavery, segregation, and ghettoization have had the collective effect of creating in the minds of many black people (African-American men) doubt concerning their human worth and dignity. To this day, the power of white Christian society to define the ultimate worth of black people and blackness has created within many black (African-Americans/ men) a doubt about their equality with whites.[197]

Without a doubt, any theology that is going to be effective and liberating for African-American men must be one that embraces the *Imago Dei*. The creation narratives in Genesis 1:27 and Genesis 2:7 provide the basis for human dignity. Human kind is a creation *ex nihilo* of God. The doctrine of creation and Judeo-Christian anthropology goes hand in hand. This biblical affirmation is the foundation of dignity and self-esteem in the family and community. The Genesis accounts says, "God saw everything that he had made and behold, it was very good."[198] Consequently, African-American men are empowered to reject any evaluation of themselves as any less of a human than anyone else. Despite the negative media images of African-American men as monstrous sub-human criminals or problems to society, they are prepared to combat the negativity mentally. In this common scenario African-American men are affirmed as somebody, regardless of employment status, economic condition, or media projections when the *Imago Dei* is acknowledged in the theological process.

---

[197] Salley, Columbus; Behm, Ronald. *What Color Is Your God?* (Downers Grove, Illinois: Intervarsity Press, 1981) Pg. 64.
[198] Genesis 1:31. KJV. Bible

## DEVELOPING A MODEL FOR LIBERATION & TRANSFORMATION

Notwithstanding what Scripture declares, Western hegemony in its alienation from God continues to deem necessary the deliberate oppression of other beings. In America, African-American men in particular still suffer from the psychological brutalities of slavery, and while African-American men are no longer physical slaves, many are still psychological slaves. And much of the oppression promulgated within the African-American community is because of the ignorance of African-American history. No longer should any church or church leadership tolerate a theology that is mainly metaphysical and abstract. To minister effectively to African-American men, The Church and its leadership must be transformative in constructing a liberating theology that intentionally seeks to remedy the dilemmas at hand; not having a theology that endears African-American men to a Christocentric perspective that is both attractive and appealing to traumatized individuals but not effective in helping remedy their realest problems. Therefore, the theological/kerygmatic community must chart a practical strategy that can move African-American men into holistic Christian living. It must begin with knowledge of the God who became incarnate in Jesus and a comprehensive awareness of the contributions of Africans to every known discipline. This will go a long way towards leading African-American men out of the abyss of inferiority; based on my research and the medical definitive causes of clinical depression, this type of information will go a long way in thwarting feelings that perpetuate trauma. The collective feelings of inferiority are integral for interpreting the attitudes and behavioral responses that are indicative of clinical depression in many African-American men. Once African-American men get in touch with their true selves, they will be able to reverse the devastating effects of oppression in America. As Na'im Akbar says:

## DEVELOPING A MODEL FOR LIBERATION & TRANSFORMATION

We can reverse the destructive effects of slavery/ (clinical depression) by looking to strengths in our past and beginning to make plans for our future. If we begin to direct our children's attention to strong images like themselves, they will grow in self-respect. We must honor and exalt our own heroes, and those heroes must be people who have done the most to dignify us (African-Americans) as a people. We must definitely avoid the psychologically destructive representations of God in a Caucasian form.[199]

In closing, I believe that The Church must consider a Womanist theology as well. I believe that a Womanist theology is necessary for African-American male reformation because, according to Raquel A. St. Clair in her book *Call and Consequences: A Womanist Reading of Mark*, "The attention given to gender issues that is evident in Womanist theology doesn't stop there. They are committed to the wholeness of entire people." She further asserts that Womanist theologians are particularly concerned with the 'isms' that oppress African-American women. "Our work masks, disentangles, and debunks religious language, symbols, doctrines and social-political structures that perpetuate the oppression of African-American women in particular, *but also African-American men, children, humanity in general*, and nature."[200] One good example of this Womanist theory at work is the Children's Defense Fund led by Marian Wright Edelman, an African-American woman; this organization has championed the causes of poverty for all children, not just African-American children. Another reason why I think Womanist theology will help bring healing for African-American men is because too often African-Americans, especially men, are too isolated and alienated in our approach to the liberation of all people. Womanist theology is expansive in its objective to fight oppression, which goes beyond the survival, liberation, and well-being of

[199] Akbar, Na'im. *Chains and Images of Psychological Slavery* (Jersey City, New Jersey: New Mind Productions, 1984) Pg. 1.
[200] St. Clair, Raquel A. *Call and Consequences: A Womanist Reading of Mark* (Minneapolis: Fortress Press, 2008) Pg. 16.

African-American women.[201] Gender, race, and class intersect and reinforce each other in the lives of African-American women; therefore, Womanist theology does not limit itself to sexism and/or "analysis of white racism" but also includes issues of class.[202] Additionally, a Womanist theological perspective is useful for other very practical reasons for African-American men suffering from clinical depression. Many African-American men who are suffering from clinical depression are being taken care of by residing with African-American women. Moreover, African-American women are more likely to be the most impacted by the mental anguish of clinically depressed African-American men. Therefore, to bring healing to the whole community, both the African-American woman and man are in need of a theological perspective that will address both of them while connecting them to others who are just like them or are going through things similar to what they are going through. I'm fully convinced that Womanist theology is a comprehensive approach to healing the whole community inclusive of men, women, and children, and all oppressed people, while working towards overcoming racism, oppression and marginalization for everyone.

If The Church is going to lead the way in transformation of African-American men in the 21st century, we must also equip and empower our laity. Findley B. Edge said:

One of the major attacks of the Reformation was centered at the point of recapturing the ministry of the laity...In the churches today the laity in the main has the attitude that the primary responsibility for ministry rests in the hands of the clergy. The layman feels that he should support the ministry and the church with his money, by attending the services, and by doing some work, primarily for and in the church. Still the layman feels that the major responsibility

---

[201] Ibid.
[202] Ibid.

for carrying out the ministry of God in the world rests with the clergy...The sharp distinction that exists today in the churches between the clergy and the laity finds no basis in the New Testament.[203]

The Church must recapture the power of the laity in order that it will become properly equipped to propagate this alternative consciousness, which is the kingdom of God. The pastor must be removed from his/her perch of exalted ineffectiveness by allowing him/her time to equip the saints, who are supposed to get the job done. One of the reasons pastors do not teach congregations effectively is that they are being burned out doing things that the congregation ought to be doing. The Church must find creative ways to free the pastor from having to deal with triviality and the marginal issues of The Church's perfunctory functions. The pastor must be able to prepare for transformative and liberating ministry that is centered on more than mitigating current injustices and work towards thwarting structural malaise. While the theology of the Jehovah's Witness is considered heretical to many mainline Christians, their methodology in mobilizing the laity is correct; the action is not in the pulpit, except as it trains other laypersons. The action is in the pew, where those who are being trained will go forth with the gospel of transformation. Everybody heads for the pulpit in many mainline Christian traditions, but no one should go up there until they have been trained to properly "equip the saints." Otherwise, they should remain in the pew in order to be trained to become an informed and prepared layperson. In retrospect, Jesus and his disciples were laypersons rather than professional clerics. Thus, we must reanalyze our understanding of how evangelism was used in Scripture. An effective ministry must have a vibrant layperson-driven evangelism component; without this evangelistic aspect, The Church cannot really become effective.

---

[203] Edge, Findley B. *A Quest for Vitality in Religion* (Nashville, TN: Broadman Press, 1963) Pg. 100.

As African-American men become more disenfranchised, The Church will definitely have to help them to overcome their historical socioeconomic, political, and sexual frustrations. Unless there is a radical change in the socioeconomic conditions of African-American men, our communities will not be safe. As the frustration levels increase within many African-American communities, the strife and hostilities could even work toward creating a police state in this country. Therefore the role of any church that ministers to African-American men in the 21$^{st}$ century must continue to sound the trumpet against the establishment that oppresses African-American men. Yes; The Church must speak against these evils that are present in the African-American community, but we must also broaden our scope in speaking and acting against evils done to any oppressed people anywhere and everywhere.

You might ask: What is The Church's potential to do all of this? Well, About 85% of African-Americans identify themselves as either fairly religious or very religious.[204] This presents the opportunity for The Church to minister to African-American men and greatly influence their thoughts and actions on many an issue. The Black Church has historically been a rock for black people, from the earliest slavery times up through Reconstruction, Jim Crow, the Civil Rights Movement era and the many crises they faced all the way up to now. The Church has been the one place, and many times the only place, that remains a potential place for healing in the community. This is an opportunity that The Church must develop in order to bring healing and empowerment to the community. Janet Taylor, MD., of Harlem Hospital says that there are some factors that contribute to positive mental health; she argues that having social support, feeling love, connecting with your physical/ spiritual self, and helping others are helpful for reducing the symptoms of

---

[204] Williams, Terrie M. *Black Pain: It Just Looks Like We're Not Hurting* (New York: Scribner Books, 2008)

depression. It is extremely important that it be known that diagnosed clinical depression has an 80% cure rate.[205] Therefore, there is no need for these men to suffer alone or in silence. Help is out there, effective help. And The Church has to become the conduit to bring that help and salvation/healing to these men. Specifically, it is vitally important that The Church positions itself to allow healing to happen by encouraging therapy and healing through both counseling and therapy sessions. That way, despite the barriers that could prohibit help and healing for the men, such as insurance and exorbitant costs for therapy, they still can seek healing. (Many of those barriers can be broken down by making men aware of the various programs that exist to assist in payment for services and encouraging them to pursue them, or pursuing Medicaid and Medicare for those who are not able to pay out of pocket nor have the proper insurance for getting assistance.)

Also, identifying professionals who could educate, train and break down the barriers of ignorance concerning the disease could be effective within a church setting. Inviting and introducing psychiatrists, psychologists, and social workers to various groups; meeting and even creating coffee hours after church; and sending emails with information and profiles of professionals and job descriptions are effective methods for informing people on these various issues. This is a pastoral response to clinical depression; therefore, I am not making any suggestions for medication because that is not the training of a pastor. Medical professionals and therapists are the appropriate people to make that kind of prognosis for those who need medication. I encourage pastors and church staff to make referrals and not try to be mental healthcare professionals themselves.

So, to be more specific, what The Church should do is create Bible classes, men's

---

[205] Ibid.

study groups, and fellowship opportunities where men can fellowship and share their emotions in a confidential setting that is non-judgmental. Furthermore, these group sessions should be very nurturing for men who are suffering from the emotional and social abuses that have been vividly described in this book. Dr. Janet Taylor too, argues that social support, feelings of well-being, and connection with physical/spiritual self encourages healing.[206] This is what I have done at Kaighn Avenue Baptist Church in Camden, New Jersey ~ create community for men to share with one another their struggles and emotions and engage in social and political reflections, while studying Scripture for reinforcement and empowerment. {In my own context of pastoring an urban African-American congregation, the opportunities I take to share with the men are every Sunday during Sunday School at 9am for one hour and a half and every 4th Saturday at 9:00am for Men's Fellowship, which is also a fellowship for the men that last one hour and a half. Various men's activities and forums are constructed to allow information, fellowship, and conversation among the men who are members of the church and within the community. These fellowships for men are formatted to be very informal, conversational, and non-confrontational. Additionally, all session workshops, discussions and plenaries are meant to be provocative on some theme that is designed to bring up conversation on a salient theme that brings insightfulness about what African-American men confront through a biblical text. I also encourage churches to have regular Men's Retreats, Men's Prayer Breakfasts, Big Brother/Little Brother outings, and Men's Celebration Days on Sunday.}

---

[206] Ibid. Pg. 262.

# <u>Appendix A</u> – <u>Teaching Theories</u>

The city of Camden is known as one of the worst cities in America. Camden is a city, based on the 2000 U.S. census, with nearly 86,000 residents, the vast majority of whom are children.[207] The poverty rate in the city is one of the highest in the area, and it is the highest by far of most municipalities in the state of New Jersey and the Delaware Valley, the region in which Camden City is located.[208] The high poverty rate and the physical of condition of the city are contributing factors to the sense of desolation in this community. The city suffers from rampant crime, high unemployment, juvenile delinquency, and the ravages of drug culture. Additional factors include disenfranchisement, and high incarceration rates particularly among African-American men.[209] Camden, like many urban areas, is struggling to deal with a disproportionate dislocation and disenfranchisement of African-American men. Too often the local culture perpetuates demonized and grotesque images of African-American men being subjectively satirized as brutish beasts. Tragically, there is a tendency to overlook this problem on the part of many citizens and see it as a concern for the government or the judicial system. Moreover, for many, even the terror of ubiquitous homicides, rampant crime, and large numbers of African-American men in prison and the correctional system have not been sufficient to bring awareness to this reality. I believe it's clear that clinical depression causes some of the high incarceration rates, low educational achievement, homicides, and violent crimes among African-American men in Camden and other cities like it.

Perhaps one of the greatest travesties concerning African-American men who

---

[207] Gillette, Howard. *Camden After The Fall: Decline and Renewal in a Post-Industrial City* (Philadelphia: University Of Pennsylvania Press, 2005) Pgs. 2-13.
[208] Ibid.
[209] Ibid.

may be suffering from undiagnosed clinical depression is that the churches they attend and want to attend throughout the nation are silent, in denial, or totally uninformed about the effects of clinical depression or its symptoms as a prognosis. One possible reason for clinical depression not being a prognosis for African-American men could be the lack of healthcare and a dearth of information concerning the disease in many African-American communities. Another reason for the lack of information concerning the disease in the African-American community could be the historically derisive treatment of African-Americans by the healthcare system in the United States. Therefore, acknowledging and properly addressing clinical depression is paramount for The Church. And though I feel that The Church should take the communal lead in advocating for African-American men who suffer from clinical depression, that does not exempt other social agencies from participating in the struggle to combat the disease as well. However, the Christian Church is vitally relevant in responding to the various nuances of African-American men suffering from mental illnesses, which are most likely undiagnosed and therefore perpetuating poor inner city African-American men foregoing medical treatment, so as far as I'm concerned the Christian Church *is* the primary, but not exclusive, focus as an agent of transformation. And some attempts to define "Church" may be inexact. The Christian Church, not just African-American churches within urban areas, is defined as a group of people summoned to live in community/fellowship with each other as they share the worship, values, morals and ethos as predicated on the Judeo-Christian principles of a total reading of the Christian Bible with Jesus the Christ in Scripture as the central figure. My extended definition of The Church is a community of people who share in community with others as they give expression to their religion and spirituality through a common ethos and genre.

The Church is well-situated to lead the charge in the fight because it functions as an institution and image of restoration and hope. Nevertheless, my contention is that depression education is the most expedient means by which to transform attitudes and cultivate behavior change. Therefore, the assumption that guides this project is that The Church can best respond to African-American men suffering from the clinical depression pandemic with education/advocacy that transforms attitudes towards African-American men in urban areas. By advocating and partnering with local churches and government agencies, it is possible to foster conditions that promote hope and help for depressed men by creating and enhancing their lives with new initiatives, social programs, support groups, and new productive ministries of social and spiritual uplift. The Church, in the perspective of this thesis, is a divinely established institution whose position is always to invite the community to engage the inveterate issues of the culture. The Church must lead as a prophetic voice and advocate for extremely vulnerable inner city African-American men. Certainly, The Church must prophetically oppose the structures and systems that impede anyone from equal participation in life the way God intended through the Holy Scriptures - the Bible. Furthermore, The Church is responsible for articulating the intent of God as it validates prophetic ministry. There is a theological imperative in prophetic ministry which presses The Church to do all it can to right wrongs and correct injustice within society.

Within many urban African-American congregations many congregants are suffering from social and economic ills, which are often compounded by disenfranchisement and severe poverty. The combination of alienation, disenfranchisement, and severe poverty renders many to suffer from vexation and frustration. The vexation, frustration, and mental anguish can promote trauma, which can lead to clinical depression. Notwithstanding, The Church must become an instrument of divine healing. The Church should be a prophetic voice and an advocate for the marginalized and the poor in society. The Church is responsible for championing justice, restoration, and wholeness as it empowers people to pick up the broken pieces of their lives. The Church is transcendent in essence and by design, ought to reflect all that is divinely good in practice. The Church should take the lead as advocate for African-American men suffering with clinical depression because these men are in need of hope. The Church is a symbol of hope; whatever is oppressive or destructive within its community should be challenged and transformed by the message, ministry, and mandate of The Church. This is the mission of The Church in every age; to bring hope and inspiration to society. It is because of this message of hope that The Church is called into action in ameliorating the social ills that surround the plight of African-American men. This hope of The Church encourages one to live in fellowship with God and others as well. The ultimate goal of the fellowship is to call the greater community to exemplify the greater good for all, especially its practitioners of the faith. Hence, there remains arguably no greater institution whereby this conviction should be taught and practiced than The Church, whose sole purpose is advocating for the outcast.

Prophetic ministry, as I understand and practice it, is the *raison d'être* of The Church. In other words, the very reason The Church exists is to engage the world's problems on behalf of those who suffer injustice. Consequently, if The Church is not engaged in fulfilling its objective as an agent of change it is ineffective. Notwithstanding, the leadership in The Church must be unequivocally committed and courageous about confronting political powers or political systems. For that reason, to be effective, the transformative leader must be prophetic, able to speak with authority and keenly aware of the issues with which one is confronted. This prophetic leader must not be beholden to political parties or political leaders; this kind of attachment will hinder their ability to speak truth to power because they will have to consider political expediency. This person must not be shackled to the past or to anything or anyone, including the church's leadership. This transformative position is a commission that calls for leaders and leadership where one who confronts the powers that be must be a champion for the cause and committed to the marginalized that are being represented. According to Walter Brueggemann, the task of prophetic ministry is to nurture, nourish, and evoke a consciousness and perception different from the consciousness and perception of the dominant culture around us.[210] The role of prophetic ministry is to rightly criticize and energize. It criticizes the injustice and social ills of society and gives voice to the wrongs that it discovers. Prophetic ministry is a catalyst for transformation. Change begins by asking whether something is imaginable, not whether it is feasible or realistic. Imagination is to precede implementation. In other words, prophetic ministry opposes the dominant culture when it is hegemonic in its composition. Along with this domination are those behaviors, which force the "others" of society to enter systems and institutions at a subordinate or subservient level. For example, African-American men suffer and silently struggle with clinical depression at subordinate and subservient levels due to an overwhelmingly broad array of factors, including overt and covert poverty, racism, injustice, unemployment, being racial profiling, incarceration at rates of genocidal magnitudes, violence and other affects in which they find themselves.

In *God's Politics: A New Vision for Faith and Politics in America,* Jim Wallis writes that prophecy is not future telling, but articulating moral truth. Prophets

---

[210] Herzog, William R. II. *The Prophetic Imagination* (The Prophetic Tradition in Biblical Leadership classroom lecture notes, Colgate Rochester; Crozer, Rochester, New York, 5-9 June 2006)

diagnose the present and point the way to a just solution. The "prophetic tradition", if practiced by all of the world's great religions, is just what is needed to open up the current political options which now are failing to offer proper influence in the context of this country's most pressing social situations.[211] Prophetic ministry confronts oppressive systems and concepts of "empire", whereby nations maneuver hegemonically unabated as they seek to perpetuate their economic and military viability. Prophetic ministry holds empires, nations, and systems accountable for their evils and injustices. Prophetic leadership is the natural corollary that is the mission of the leader or preacher of a congregation of believers; the pastor and leaders of the congregation should inspire change for the community to embody transformative leadership. Furthermore, the leadership must engage comprehensively a ministry that pursues the agenda of justice for the whole of the world through the church. The connection and collaboration of prophetic ministry and transformative ministry energizes as it empowers and informs, particularly those in the Reign of God, to boldly proclaim the universal dignity, worth and value of God's creation. This is the energy that Jesus of the Lukan Gospel experiences as he declares, immediately before radically dismantling the world and its systems, that "the Spirit of the Lord is upon me and has anointed me to preach the gospel."[212] By not being engaged in such work, the church compromises its role and becomes irrelevant because it is inconsistent with the divine purpose.

Consequently, The Church is to be the institution that leads the charge and pushes for radical change for acceptance and the inclusion and enfranchisement of African-American men. But The Church can't do it all; the government has a big

---

[211] Wallis, Jim. *God's Politics: A New Vision for Faith and Politics in America* (New York: HarperCollins Publishers, 2005) Pg. 72.
[212] Luke 4:18. KJV Bible.

role to play in this change. It must be in covenant with The Church and its leadership when it comes to this. Government must be on the front line of the amelioration of African-American men, and thus should be pushing for radical change too. This radical push is to be conceptualized through the dynamics of transformative leadership. Transformative leadership combined with a prophetic mission/ ministry for the greater community, as it formulates, is the desire to move a person or group physically, spiritually, socially, psychologically and economically from one point to another point, always in a positive proclivity. Transformative leadership consists of processes that offer a vision that depicts what things should be like. Within this context, transformative leadership is radical in its essence. It is inconsistent with the norm, which validates the ramifications of the affects of shame, stigma, guilt, disgust, frustration, alienation, racism, and other structures that impede one from equitable participation in society and promotes xenophobic and racist attitudes towards African-American men and their families. Can the dynamics of transformative leadership, however one defines them, change a person's or an institution's posture toward African-American men's issues with clinical depression? If transformation and change is to occur through the interconnectivity of education, mission and outreach, how will it be designed? (This book concludes with some suggestions for the transformative leader who is directing a prophetic ministry for African-American men suffering with clinical depression.)

Transformative leadership serves as a catalyst, which promotes awareness concerning the plight of African-American men. If this leadership is practiced by the church and accompanied by appropriate government intervention, social change is inevitable. If both entities aggressively push for changes that debunk misinformed theories and images of African-American men, change is possible.

One such erroneous theory is that African-American men are inveterate criminals. Many others believe African-American men only want to sell drugs and commit crime; therefore, they deserve to be incarcerated without any further consideration. The latter assertion, that African-American men should be incarcerated, is a position adopted by many churches, including some African-American congregations, pastors and church leaders. This shortsighted perspective forestalls the church from engaging in advocating for African-American men in crisis. Some misinformed circles actually believe that the "War on Drugs" has brought a near end to crime. However, the necessary transformation will occur only if educational efforts are intentional and consistent. A greater challenge, however, is encouraging leaders to enter into a general and objective dialogue concerning the plight of African-American men. The relationship between crime and African-American men needs to be addressed more thoroughly. So basically I'm saying that transformation is necessary not only for many black men, but for The Church, the government, and many folks in our society too. And since transformation begins with oneself, the practitioners of transformative leadership must themselves first be transformed.

The context of ministry is a determining factor as to which type of leadership model is most effective. There is no singular or "one size fits all" definition of transformative leadership. One thing's for certain: The transformer must embrace the vision for transformation wholeheartedly. The process of transformative leadership involves moving further into the reign of God, and leadership that is in transformation naturally seeks to cultivate that transformation in others. Mahatma Gandhi was quoted once to have said, "We must be the change we wish to see in the world."[213] Gandhi's statement encourages transformative leaders to begin where they are; amid the religious and theological communities, throughout the local and geographical sphere, permeating the social and political systems. All levels of leadership and policy-makers are to be visibly imbued and influenced in order for others to readily be encouraged to participate in transformation. It is imperative that one who seeks to transform the situation understands the resources and principles of transformative leadership within their context. Due to the substantial volume of information on transformation leadership, I will briefly draw conclusions from some of those relevant models of transformative leadership.

James M. Kouzes and Barry Posner, the authors of a significant book on leadership entitled *The Leadership Challenge*, do not call the prevailing principles which make up an exemplary leadership paradigm "transformative leadership." However, they do offer resources and principles essential for good leadership. I will examine Kouzes and Posner's concepts on exemplary leadership as a guide for elaboration and discussion. Contained in *The Leadership Challenge* is a statement that gives credence to these leadership principles as being transformative in essence:

Leadership that focuses on committing and transforming style and perception are what leadership scholars have called transformational leadership. Transformational leadership occurs when, in their interaction, people raise one another to higher levels of motivation and morality. Their purposes, which might have started out as separate but relaxed, as in the case of transactional leadership, become fused. Notwithstanding transforming leadership ultimately becomes moral in that it raises the level of human conduct and ethical aspiration of both the leader and the led,

---

[213] Herzog, William R. II. *The Prophetic Imagination* (The Prophetic Tradition in Biblical Leadership classroom lecture notes, Colgate Rochester Crozer Divinity School, Rochester, New York, 5-9 June 2006)

thereafter it has a transforming effect on both.[214]

In the book, there are multiple models of leadership being marketed. No singular model is a panacea for all situations and leadership is situational. However, there are elements of leadership that appear to be essential to most if not all models. *The Leadership Challenge* articulates some definitive components essential to all leadership. Although the actual words "transformation" and "transformative leadership" are not used as the official descriptive terms for defining models of leadership, elements consistent with my contextual definition are present within the descriptions. For instance, in most leadership models, there are elements of trust, credibility, integrity, morality, and engaging others. And it is a fact that those who give leadership must trust those who lead. Additionally though, there is the element of Modeling; one who leads, in any leadership style, must be able to demonstrate one's leadership philosophy. And Vision; setting or prognosticating the outcome or future is essential to all leadership styles and paradigms. James Kouzes and Barry Posner delineate a model of leadership that consists of five elements or five practices of exemplary leadership.[215] Briefly, exemplary leadership models the way; inspires a shared vision; challenges the process; enables others to act; and encourages the heart.[216] My point is: If these components are infused into the process designed to address the crisis of clinic depression among the African-American men as a modality offered to effectuate change, transformation is inevitable. (A "helping hand" in designing that construct or model is what this book is meant to offer; not the total answer, but simply a pre-model for ministering to clinically depressed African-American men.)

---

[214] Kouzes, James M.; Posner, Barry Z. *The Leadership Challenge* (San Francisco: Jossey-Bass, publisher, 2003) Pg. 153.
[215] Ibid. Pgs. 12-22.
[216] Ibid. Pgs. 12-22.

An effective model consists of a process that is able to secure knowledge and facts and then focus on the means whereby the resources of transformative leadership are able to cultivate a culture for change. Modeling the way, according to James Kouzes and Barry Posner, means one discovering one's own voice for leadership in order to say what is meant. This stage incorporates the leader being able to clarify his or her values and being able to express those values. It also concerns the leader possessing strong beliefs about matters of principle, having an unwavering commitment to a clear set of values, and being passionate about one's cause.[217] (Additionally, in this section on the model of leadership, there is a focus on the leader finding his or her voice for leadership. The exemplary leader is able to speak from his or her core of beliefs. Those who are being led must know it is the leader's voice and vision they are hearing.[218] This involves the transformative leader believing in their message and vision; people who are being led must understand that the transformative leader really believes in the cause being framed before them.)

Notwithstanding, in *church leadership,* Lovett Weems believes that behavior is the key to credibility. "People perceive us", writes Weems, "as doing what we say we are going to do. Predictability has become a key to trust."[219] Parenthetically, Lovett Weem's model of leadership also proposed many characteristic traits of leadership, a few of which are vision, team, culture and integrity.[220] Leadership should inspire a shared vision that involves envisioning the future and enlisting others. One must be able to look toward the future; seeing things not as they are, but rather, as one imagines them. The exemplary leader is one who is able "to see

---

[217] Ibid. Pgs. 43-60.
[218] Ibid.
[219] Weems, Lovett H., Jr. *Church Leadership Vision, Team, and Integrity* (Nashville, TN: Abingdon Press, 1993) Pg. 127.
[220] Ibid.

something out ahead," as vague as it might appear from a distance. Exemplary leaders imagine that extraordinary feats are possible and that the ordinary could be transformed into something noble.[221]

Vision is essential to every leadership style. It assists in defining and articulating the direction to be traversed. Visioning keeps people and organizations on a predetermined path. Visioning allows people and organizations to embrace a realistic ideal of hope for the future. If transformative leadership is offered as a type of resolve for behavioral change among the church and government leaders, efforts must intensify. Lovett Weems writes:

Where there is a powerful and compelling vision, people look to the future for hope. Such a concept can lift people out of their ordinary and conventional ways of thinking and working. It gives a boost to morale and a lift to the spirit.[222]

In order to facilitate change within the religious community concerning prejudice and preconceived notions that surround African-American men's clinical depression, it is essential to challenge the process. Challenging the process means being inventive and creative while standing up for ones' beliefs. Oftentimes the challenge is to be radical in one's thinking. In the context of assessing clinical depression among African-American men, challenging the process is about discovering and planting new partnerships, creative programs and ministries. It requires being innovative. Innovation requires more listening and communication than routine work. Leadership that guides a change must therefore establish more relationships, connect with more sources of information, and get out and walk around more frequently. This is connected to the last two parts of the suggested

---

[221] Ibid. Kouzes. Pg. 191.
[222] Ibid. Weems. Pg. 62.

principles for exemplary leadership as well; enabling others to act and encouraging the heart. This consists of the leader projecting a vision plan that can be fully embraced by those being led. It is sharing one's destiny and not designing in a vacuum. Enabling others and encouraging the heart is the process of developing and discovering others, their dreams, their aspirations, and what is appealing to them.[223]

Due to the nature of clinical depression and the fact that this disease could possibly affect African-Americans men disproportionately, there is a need for those who deal with African-American men to be properly trained concerning clinical depression and the plight of African-American men. Furthermore, it is the clergy who provide leadership in what has historically been the most influential institution in the African-American community; The Church. Many clergy are either ignorant or misinformed concerning the severity and prevalence of the disease. Many pastors and congregations are living under the misconception that their congregations are immune to clinical depression, or that the disease is something that the church should not engage, while others believe it is just a spiritual problem that is caused by a demonic oppression and should be exorcised - or "cased" out by the clergy. Notwithstanding, if the pastor or the clergy and the leadership of the congregation do not see clinical depression as a serious condition, nothing can happen to transform the condition of African-American men who are suffering. It is extremely important that the Christian Church take interest in the condition of African-American men. The response of The Church toward acceptance of the presence of clinical depression among African-American men is based upon an articulated vision of clinical depression education and treatment, which should be held by both the clergy and the parishioners.

---

[223] Ibid.

Simultaneously, there is a need for local government to be educated as to the significance of clinical depression in African-American men. Local government, which includes health departments and elected officials, are postured at junctures for advocacy to bring awareness, education and opportunities to fight the shame, stigma, and other negative attitudes associated with clinical depression. For instance, in Camden, New Jersey, specifically the congregation of Kaighn Avenue Baptist Church, 28% of the church's congregants are African-American men. This congregation is in a very depressed urban area in Southern New Jersey where unemployment for African-American men is above 50%.[224] Joblessness and poverty are among the highest in the nation in Camden, one of New Jersey's poorest cities, though New Jersey itself is ironically one of the wealthiest states in America. The African-American men in Camden, N.J., like in many other wealthy states in this country with extremely poor despots of blacks in them or near them, are under conditions rife for suffering from clinical depression and it cannot be overstated that our local government must be a part of the process if resolve is to be brought to these men. The government possesses funds that can be distributed for preventive literature, hand bills, public announcements, workshops, summits, partnering, and other creative and diverse methods geared to combating the disease and misinformation. In some instances, it is at the local government level that legislation may need to be challenged or changed. As The Church enters into dialogue with government, it must have the opportunity to be involved at the funding level. (An authentic example of the role that government can adopt in the clinical depression struggle is progressing at the time of the writing of this book; I am working on the State of New Jersey's Safe Streets & Neighborhoods Oversight Committee as an advocate for men who have been incarcerated and at-risk men in

---

[224] Gillette, Howard. *Camden After The Fall: Decline and Renewal in a Post-Industrial City* (Philadelphia, PA: Philadelphia Press, 2005) Pgs. 2-13.

the urban areas of New Jersey, whom are overwhelmingly African-American and Hispanic. Also I am organizing the Men's Ministry of Kaighn Avenue Baptist Church to begin a community advocacy ministry to minister to men who are members of the congregation and the community. This ministry is for men in Camden County halfway houses and in Camden County jails. There are many tangible opportunities for local government here in Camden, and local governments in every other city and county, to both learn and assist in this effort if only they would to a substantial enough degree.)

Another group that should be educated is the people most vulnerable to men highly likely to suffer from clinical depression. In this group are wives, girlfriends, mothers, children, family members, co-workers, and friends. Indeed there are subtle nuances that accompany each at-risk group. However, the named categories themselves are sufficient to describe who are at-risk and how and why they are at risk. The goal is to create support for men suffering from clinical depression, so the church should encourage families and friends of these men to identify the symptoms of clinical depression. *All* those who are "suffering with" clinical depression need to be educated as to the disease and how to combat this mental illness. A concern of mine and a concern of psychologists who study clinical depression is that African-American men who suffer from clinical depression will be seen as "soft", "weak" and as being "effeminate" by those close to them.[225] Clinical depression carries, to many men but also to those around them, a double stain - the stigma of mental illness and also the stigma of "feminine" emotionality. There is an imperative that some institution(s) become a voice to counteract this kind of misinformation concerning clinical depression. My belief is that the local

[225] Real, Terrance. *I Don't Want To Talk About It: The Secret Legacy of Make Depression* (New York: Scribner Books, 1997) Pgs. 38-41.

church, especially urban congregations, must become institutions that do this.

Really, The Church has to be willing to listen, educate, and empower the whole community on clinical depression. In the context of the African-American community, there are people of influence of who operate in non-official roles and outside the political sphere. These people are not clergy, pastors, or community leaders. Notwithstanding, these people are respected people of influence and power brokers within the community. Their voices resonate from beauty salons, barbershops and other neighborhood enterprises. These people are men and women who are respected community leaders, grandparents, celebrities, rap artists, and news anchorpersons. Thus, the leadership that The Church must facilitate on clinical depression is not simply political leadership. The Church needs to lead in building partnerships and coalitions for advocating for African-American men. This leadership would include developing a viable plan to become a resource for elected officials serving at the state, local, and community levels. This leadership must be inclusive of educational institutions, faith communities, the Urban League, and the NAACP; every organization that could be an instrument in engaging the community concerning the plight of African-American men must be consulted.

Again, clinical depression can be treated if properly diagnosed. If the condition of many urban African-American men could be reassessed and properly analyzed by asking why are so many African-American men incarcerated, victims of homicides, and disenfranchised within society, I believe that the assessment in and of itself promotes the idea that many African-American men are suffering with undiagnosed and untreated clinical depression. But the question still remains as to what particular models of education would help better understand and promote clinical depression education amongst African-Americans. David H. Kelsey describes two models of education, and in my opinion it is under these models of education that knowledge, revelation, "good" research and professional education are to be understood. Upon critical analysis, both models could be used to infer theories and methodologies, which can assist in bringing clarity to the issue of clinical depression. Also, I contend that the models of education he proposes, if properly understood, are capable of providing resources for understanding the need for clinical depression education at a religious/spiritual level and at the research level. According to Kelsey, in his book *Between Athens and Berlin: The Theological Debate*, theological education is framed within the models termed "Athens" and "Berlin".[226] The Athens model of theological education is based on schooling in ancient Greek culture. Athens is a type of schooling for which *paideia* is the heart of education. *Paideia*, in Greek, is the process of "culturing" the soul; using schooling as "character formation". It is the oldest type of education found in Christianity.[227] The Athens model has long exercised authority over Christian understanding of both Christianity and education. Werner Jaeger, the foremost historian of paideia, claims that this model of education "can be pursued through the Middle Ages and {that} from the Renaissance the line leads straight back to the Christian humanism of the father of the 4th century A.D." [228] The goal of paideia is knowledge of "good" itself, which requires conversion, a turning around of the soul, from preoccupation.[229] Education as paideia is defined as inquiry into a single, underlying principle of all virtues and their essences. To be shaped by excellence, is simply to know the "good".[230] The teacher cannot teach paideia; all the teacher can do is provide the student indirect assistance and demonstrate the intellectual and moral discipline that will capacitate the student for the student's

[226] Ibid. Kelsey
[227] Ibid.
[228] Ibid. Pg. 7.
[229] Ibid. Pg. 9.
[230] Ibid.

own good.[231] Going through multiple changes historically, the education model of Athens and the ideal of paideia, in the thought of many scholars, emerged as an integral part of Christianity.[232] In essence, the Christian model is simply a theological education where the goal is knowledge of "good" and correctively forming a person's soul to be holy.[233]

The Berlin model of education emerged in 1810, when the newly founded University of Berlin decided to add a faculty of theology.[234] One of the models that came from this school of theology was the binary model. This binary model stresses the interconnected importance of two different enterprises. The goals of the University were to teach students how to do research and how to master the truth about whatever subject is studied. This model was later known as a scientific model of doing effect research. Due to the level of importance placed on research, the Berlin model stood in contrast to the Athens model. The Athens model gave room for "revelation" and "intuitiveness"; in contrast, the Berlin model sincerely questioned whether a theological faculty would compromise its objective. Where the Athens model survived the Enlightenment Era without major deviations in its philosophy, the Berlin model strived to reshape education along the Enlightenment principles.[235] The Berlin model is binary because it is concerned with being applicable to a research institution and a teaching institution. The Athens model dominated all of the arts and sciences until the emergence of the Berlin model. What the philosopher Plato had been to Athens, Friedrich Schleiermacher was to Berlin. Both postulated their influence on the respective models of education.[236]

---

[231] Ibid.
[232] Ibid. Pg. 10. Kelsey
[233] Ibid. Pg. 11.
[234] Ibid.
[235] Ibid.
[236] Ibid. Pgs. 6-22. Kelsey

Hence, I believe both models are essential for the purpose of this projected effort. The Athens type is unavoidably engaged in self-conscious culture transaction with its host culture.[237] For the Berlin model, theological education is a movement from data to theory and from application of theory to practice.[238] Therefore, my concurrence rests somewhere between Athens and Berlin. The Athens model is critical since this thesis is theological and meant for a practical ministry within the context of an urban congregation serving African-American men suffering with clinical depression, and yet, the Berlin model is equally important since this thesis is heavily dependent on the validity of research. So for the purposes set forth, we would do good to combine both these models. In addition, as we move from models of education, let us see what research tells us about the history of depression.

---

[237] Ibid.
[238] Ibid.

# Appendix B – The History of Clinical Depression

We've all heard of terms like *melancholia* and *depression* and their many cognates; over the last two millennia there have literally been thousands of ways of referring to a number of different mental states in the Western world. At any particular time during these many centuries, the terms commonly used might have denoted a disease; a troublesome condition of sufficient severity and duration to be conceived of as a clinically defined malady; or it might have been referred to as one of a cluster of symptoms that were thought to constitute a disease. These symptoms might have been used to indicate a mood or an emotional state of some duration that's perhaps troublesome and certainly unusual and yet not pathological, or a disease. Many of these symptoms have referred to a temperament or type of character involving a certain emotional tone and disposition. The symptoms of depression are an onerous malady that for much of human history was totally indescribable by vocabulary. Moreover, many symptoms of what we now know to be clinical depression are indicative of a mood or psychophysical reality which can last for a short duration or for a lifetime. However, the most visible condition brought on by depression was unusual mental states, which range over a far wider spectrum than that covered by the term "disease".

As a mood, affect, or emotion, the experience of being "down" or depressed has probably been as well known to our species as any of the many other human feelings. The wide range of terms and the emotional variations to which they refer have reflected matters at the very heart of being human: experiencing melancholy, feeling blue, unhappy, being dispirited, discouraged, disappointed, dejected, despondent, and despairing. All humanity experiences emotions from discouragement, material loss, interpersonal rejection, separation, death, sorrow, emotional brokenness, dejection, etc. We also acknowledge many aspects of such affective experiences as being within the normal range, however unusual or dismayed.[239] To be in a state of melancholy or depression is not necessarily to be mental ill or in a pathological state. There are varying degrees of severity and duration where depressed states are viewed as pathological conditions and even then the affective state is usually accompanied by other symptoms before being so judged.[240] The latter condition - the pathological state - constitutes the focus of this study, if you will. Its vital roots are grounded in the history of medicine; befitting since this thesis approaches depression as a clinical condition. This study will chart the history of depression as a clinical phenomenon and examine how this disease has affected African-American men.

By choosing to focus on depression as a clinical condition, we are immediately faced with the issue of whether it is a disease or some other sort of assemblage of signs and symptoms. Thus, it became necessary to address the evolving history of the concept of disease to consider the question of disease vs. clinical syndrome, and to weigh the issues involved in disease vs. illness. It is important to trace the changes in clinical content, whether disease or syndrome. Then, what relationship did these conditions have to symptoms, temperaments, sustained feeling states, and passing frames of mind? This is where the history of the passions and the emotions becomes relevant. The history of explanations of this disease is crucial because it helps to explain how depression has been recognized and treated historically. Thus, there is a need to study the terminology and the history of how clinical depression and those suffering with the disorder have been acknowledged therapeutically.

---

[239] Strock, Margaret. *Depression*, NIH Publication No. 04- 3561, National Institute of Mental Health, National Institutes of Health, U.S. Department Of Health and Human Services, Bethesda, MD. (2004)
[240] Ibid.

## Origins of the Terminologies for Depression

*Melancholia* was the Latin transliteration of the Greek word "μελαλχολία" which in ancient Greece usually meant a mental disorder involving prolonged fear and depression.[241] It sometimes merely meant "biliousness" and along with its cognates, was sometimes used in popular speech "to denote crazy or nervous conduct".[242] This term, in turn, translated from Greek into Latin as "atra bilis" and into English as "black bile".[243] Early in the acknowledgement of the disease, the black bile was thought to be the crucial etiological factor in *melancholia*. There were many other disorders believed to come from the black bile. The various forms of *melancholia* and its cognates, taken with relatively little change from the Latin, began to appear in English writings in the 14th century. Terms such as *malencolye*, *malancoli*, *malecolie*, *melancholie*, *melancholy* and others, with only slight variations in spelling, emerged as synonyms for *melancholia* early in Western history. *Melancholie* in the 16th century and *melancholy* by the beginning of the 17th century became common English equivalent terms to *melancholia* for naming the disease, as did nearly identical terms in other vernacular languages; and these terms were also frequently used to mean the black bile.[244] Moreover, in the 17th and 18th centuries *melancholia* seems to have been the vernacular throughout many parts of Western Europe for naming the disease we call *depression*.[245] Almost any state of sorrow, dejection, or despair beyond somber and fashionable sadness was described in the context of the word we now use to denote *depression* today.

*Depression* is a relatively new term for feeling "down" or "blue". This term

---

[241] Jackson, Stanley W. *Melancholia and Depression: From Hippocratic Times to Modern Times* (New Haven: Connecticut, 1986) Pg. 4.
[242] Ibid.
[243] Ibid.
[244] Ibid.
[245] Ibid.

originates from the Latin terms *de* (which means down from) and *premere* (to press down) and *deprimere* (to press down) and thus carrying the meanings from these Latin terms of pressing down, being pressed down, and being brought down in status or fortune, this term and its cognates came into use in English during the 17th century.[246] During this same period there were instances of the terms being used to illuminate what was called "depression of spirits" or "dejection."[247] During the 18th century, the connection between *depression* and what was termed *melancholia* became prominent. Samuel Johnson, author of the English Dictionary, later provided us with the meaning of *melancholy* being defined as "a kind of madness, in which the mind is always fixed on one object....a disease, supposed to proceed from a redundance of black bile; but it is better known to arise from too heavy and too viscid blood: its cure is in evacuation, nervous medicines, and powerful stimuli."[248] In 1725, Richard Blackmore mentioned the possibility of "being depressed into deep sadness and melancholy, or elevated into lunacy and distraction."[249] Robert Whytt in 1764 associated "depression of mind" with low spirits, hypochondriasis, and *melancholy.*[250] David Daniel Davis in 1806 translated, from the French of 1801, Philippe Pinel's *Treatise on Insanity,* rendering *l'abattement* as "depression of spirits" and *habitude d'abattement et d consternation* as "habitual depression and anxiety."[251] John Haslam in 1808 referred to "those under the influence of the depressing passion."[252] And Samuel Tuke in 1813 included under *melancholia* "all cases...in which the disorder is chiefly marked by depression of mind."[253]

---

[246] Ibid. Pg. 5.
[247] Ibid.
[248] Ibid. Pg. 144.
[249] Ibid.
[250] Ibid.
[251] Ibid.
[252] Ibid.
[253] Ibid.

The 19th century saw an increasingly frequent use of the term *depression* and its cognates in literary context to mean depression of spirits, *melancholia*, and *melancholy*. The use of the same terms in medical contexts gradually increased those descriptive accounts of *melancholic* disorders denoting affect or mood; the terms had not yet been acquired to represent a formal diagnostic category or any kind of status for diagnostic study of the disease. In the middle of the century, Wilhelm Griesinger introduced the term *states of mental depression* (*Die psychischen Depresionzustande*) as a synonym for *melancholia (Melancholie)* while using *depression* and its kin to distinguish or indicate affect or mood in the manner just mentioned.[254] During the latter half of the 19th century the descriptive use of the term *depression* to describe the affect becoming increasingly common though the basic diagnostic term was still usually *melancholia* or *melancholy.*[255] Much like Gresinger, Daniel Hake Tuke, in his *Dictionary of Psychological Medicine in 1892,* listed "mental depression" as a synonym for *melancholia* and defined "nervous depression" as "a term applied sometimes to a morbid fancy or melancholy of temporary duration"[256] but dealt with clinical states of dejection under *melancholia.*[257]It was in the 1880's in the psychoses section of his *Lehrbuch* that Emil Karaepelin began using the term *depressive insanity* (*depressive Wahnsinn*) to name one of the categories of insanity, and he included *depressive form* (*depressive Form*) as one of the categories of insanity and as one of the categories of paranoia (*Verrucktheit*); but he continued to employ *melancholia,* and subtypes thereof, in a manner consistent with his times and to use the term *depression* mainly to describe affect.[258] Parenthetically, he considered the

---

[254] Griesinger, Wilhelm. *Die Pathologie und Therapie der psychisen Krankbeiten* (Stuttgart: Adolph Krabbe, 1845 newer translation, 1972) Pgs. 152-208.
[255] Ibid. Pgs. 12-80.
[256] Ibid. Pgs. 152-186.
[257] Ibid.
[258] Ibid. Pg. 6.

melancholies to be forms of mental depression or *Psychische Depression*, which is Griesinger's term.[259] In addition, in 1899 Emil Kraepelin introduced the term *manic-depressive insanity* as a diagnostic term.[260] Since that time some form or variant of the term *depression* has had a prominent place in most nosological schemes for mental disorders. Adolf Meyer may have furthered the trend away from the use of the term *melancholia* and towards the use of *depression*. The report of a discussion in 1904 indicates that he was "desirous of eliminating the term melancholia, which implied knowledge of something that we did not possess....If, instead of melancholia, we applied the term depression to the whole class, it would designate in an unassuming way exactly what was meant by the common use of the term melancholia."[261]

Furthermore, as indicated, the term *depression* and its cognates were increasingly found in psychiatric classifications toward the end of the 19th century, and yet the basic diagnostic term for dejected states still tended to be *melancholia*. Moreover, with the emergence of the category of manic-depressive disease, the term *melancholia* became much less prominent, although it continued to be used in the form of *involutional melancholia*. Thus the latter diagnostic term has since disappeared as a distinct disorder, reappeared, and then disappeared again. (The term *melancholia* has recently emerged again, this time as a subtype of the major depressive episode in the newest classificatory system. This designation has the implication of a more severe form of depression and is characterized by symptoms much like those of the earlier categorizations of endogenous depression.)

---

[259] Jackson, Stanley W. *Melancholia and Depression: From Hippocratic Times to Modern Time* (New Haven: Connecticut, 1986)
[260] Ibid.
[261] Meyer, Adolf. *The Collected Papers of Adolf Meyer*, ed. Eunice E. Winters, 4 vols. (Baltimore: The John Hopkins Press, 1951) 2:568.

## **Various Theories on Depression**
### The Black Bile Theory

As previously noted, the term *melancholia* has its origins in the term "black bile" and it was used to literally mean the black bile of the body as well as to name a disease. The black bile concept enmeshed in the context of the humoral theory, which for two thousand years was the central explanation for dealing with the disease. The black bile, as it was called, was considered to be the fundamental element in the pathogenesis of *melancholia*. The notion of bodily humors as crucial elements in health and disease was a familiar one by the time of Hippocrates in the latter part of the 5th century B.C.[262] But the bringing together of the four humors - blood, yellow bile, phlegm, and black bile - in the theory that was to be known as *humoralism* probably did not occur until they were so presented in the Hippocratic work, *Nature of Man*:

The notion of the humours as such comes from empirical medicine. The notion of the tetrad, the definition of health as the equilibrium of the different parts, and sickness as the disturbance of this equilibrium, are Pythagorean contributions (which were taken up by Empedocles). The notion that in the course of the seasons each of the four substances in turn gains the ascendancy seems to be purely Empedocles. But the credit for combining all these notions in one system, and thereby creating the doctrine of humoralism which was to dominate the future, is no doubt due the powerful writer who composed the first... [Nature of Man]. This system included ... also the doctrine of the qualities that Philistion handed down to us - first, in groups of two, forming a link between the humours and the seasons, later also appearing singly and connecting the humours with the Empedocles primary elements. From this the author of ... [Nature of Man] evolved the following schema, which was to remain in force for more than two thousand years.[263]

Indeed as early as with the Pythagoreans, the four seasons had been matched

---

[262] Ibid. Pg. 7.
[263] Ibid.

with the Four Ages of Man, the latter being counted either as boyhood, youth, manhood or old age; or alternatively, as youth till the age of twenty, prime until about forty, decline until about sixty, and after that comes antiquation. A connection could therefore be established without much ado between the Four Humours (and later the Four Temperaments) and the Four Ages of Man - a connexion which held good for all time and which was to be of fundamental significance in the future development of both speculation and imagery. [264]

While the black bile was apparently not established as one of the four natural humors until its appearance as such in the *Nature of Man,* it was considered a noxious degeneration of the yellow bile, or alternatively, of the blood; perhaps even in pre-Hippocratic works thought to be earlier than *Nature of Man* there were at times two or three or four humors, but the black bile was not among them.[265] Sometimes blood but more commonly bile and phlegm were mentioned, with the usually clear implication that this bile was the yellow bile.[266] Along with the emergence of the balanced quartet of humors in the *Nature of Man,* the black bile seems to have graduated from the status of toxic product to join the yellow bile, blood, and phlegm as another basic natural ingredient in the body. Within this theory, various environmental influences and foodstuff came to be connected with formation, and with normal and abnormal proportions or amounts in the body. In its status as merely a pathogenic agent, and not yet a cardinal humor with both normal and pathological roles, in the 5th century B.C. the black bile "was held responsible for a great variety of diseases ranging from headache, vertigo,

[264] Hippocrates. *Works of Hippocrates, trans.* and ed. W. H. S. Jones and E. T. Withington, 4 vols. (Cambridge: Harvard University Press, 1923-1931) I: lviii; W. H. S. Jones. *Malaria and Greek History* (Manchester: The University Press, 1909) Pg. 100.
[265] Klibansky, Raymond; Panofsky, Erwin; Saxl, Fritz. *Saturn and Melancholy: Studies in the History of Natural Philosophy, Religion and Art* (New York: Basic Books, 1964) Pg. 8.
[266] Ibid. Pg. 8.

paralysis, spasms, epilepsy, and other mental disturbances, from quartan fever to disease of the kidney, liver, and spleen."[267] Although, in contrast to yellow bile, phlegm, and blood, it is difficult to reconcile the black bile with any known substance today, Sigerist suggested that:

In this as in other cases the Greeks gastric ulcers is black, as sometimes do patients with carcinoma of the stomach vomit the substances. A form of malaria is still known as "blackwater fever" because the urine as a result of acute intravascular hemolysis suddenly becomes very dark, if not black at least mahogany-colored. Similar observation may have led to the assumption that ordinary yellow bile through corruption could become black and that this black bile caused diseases, notably the "black disease" named melancholy.[268]

Variant forms of black bile were said to exist, and in light of frequent references to it in the medical literature of the Middle Ages and the Renaissance, one of these variants merits some consideration here. In addition to the natural black bile that had its place in health and caused *melancholic* disease when in excess, there was a second type that was known by many names: *unnatural melancholy, adust melancholy, melancholia adusta, burnt choler,* and *burnt black bile.* Eventually Galen made the assertion that the combustion of yellow bile provokes violent delirium in the presence or absence of fever, because it occupies the substance of the brain itself.[269] Subsequently, in discussing *melancholia,* he argued that some cases of the *melancholic* disease might be caused by a black bile "produced by intense local heat which burns the yellow bile or the thicker and darker blood."[270] Additionally, in his other work *One the Natural Faculties,* he referred to natural and unnatural forms of black bile, the latter being the result of "combustion caused

---

[267] Sigerist, Henry. E. *A History of Medicine,* 2 vol. (New York: Oxford University Press, 1951-1961) 2: 320.
[268] Ibid.
[269] Galen. *On the Usefulness of the Parts of the Body,* trans. and ed. Margaret T. May, 2 vols. (Ithaca: Cornell University Press, 1968) 1:232
[270] Ibid. Pg. 88.

by abnormal heat."[271] Many physicians of the time believed that natural black bile was one of the four basic humors that was sometimes derived from foodstuff and merely present and sometimes as thick and cold residue derived from the blood by a process of chilling, and of unnatural black bile or *melancholia adusta*, as formed by the corruption, overheating or burning of yellow bile.[272] The assertion was then pointed out by many other physicians that these two forms of black bile with roots in process of chilling and overheating are vaguely reminiscent of the cold and hot qualities in the black bile mentioned in a seminal work of the time, *Problemata*.[273] Increasingly the idea of an unnatural black bile, or *adust melancholy*, was developed to the point where a process of burning or combustion could affect any one of the four natural humors and so lead to the formation of burnt or adust* black bile. Eventually it became common to think of there being potentially four types of this adust black bile, each corresponding to one of the natural humors. Several of the causes suggested for such a process included improper diets, physiological disorders, and immoderate passions. The burning process would lead to a hot *adust melancholy*; cooling would eventually result in cold *adust melancholy*, which resembled natural black bile in its appearance and effects.

## The Six Non-Naturals

In ancient medicine the term "non-natural" was used to refer to a group of acquired environmental factors. Usually six in number, the careful management of these factors was believed to be crucial to health in the sense referred to as being *hygiene,* and any of which could cause disease if imbalance or disproportion of any

---

[271] Galen. *On the Natural Facilities,* trans. Arthur John Brock (Cambridge: Harvard University Press, 1963) Pg. 213.
[272] Jackson, Stanley, W. *Melancholia and Depression: From Hippocratic Times to Modern Times* (New Haven: Yale University Press, 1986) Pg. 10.
[273] Ibid.
*There is a difference between "adusta" and "adust": the permutations of the word.

of the factors existed. These were distinguished from the *seven naturals (innate)* which were the factors of normal function and constituted the basic science of ancient medicine: the elements, the temperaments, the humors, the parts of the body, the faculties, the function and the spirits. These naturals were innate constitutional factors that might be disturbed in disease, or the disturbance of which, particularly the humors, might be crucial in the pathogenesis of a disease. The non-natural was also prominent from the *contra-naturals*, which were the putative causes of disease in usual sense of the term "pathology". The six things known as non-naturals were usually air, exercise and rest, sleep and wakefulness, food and drink, excretion and retention of superfluities, and the passions or perturbations of the soul. The very doctrine of the non-naturals could be stated as: "…there are six categories of factors that operatively determine health or disease, depending on the circumstance of their use or abuse, to which human beings are unavoidably exposed in the course of daily life". Management of the regimen of the patient, that is, of his involvement with these six sets of factors, was for centuries the physician's most important task. [274] Listed by Galen in his *Ars Medica,* this scheme became a standard and significant part of later versions of Galenic medicine. The term "non-naturals" came into common use only in the wake of Latin translation of Arabic works largely based on Galen. However, the term was used in works on the pulse by Galen, who seemed to imply that both the term and the classification of six non-natural factors antedated him.[275]

The non-naturals continued to receive significant attention in medical works well into the 18th century, and eventually concerns about such matter became the physical and moral (psychological) hygiene of more recent times. The doctrine

---

[274] Ibid. Pg. 11.
[275] Ibid.

ranked alongside the humoral theory as a significant system of thought for the explanation of both health and disease, but it remained in active use well beyond the demise of the humoral theory. The non-naturals were frequently given careful attention in considering the genesis of *melancholia* and in outlining therapeutic plans for *melancholic* patients. The doctrine, within these categories of the passions or perturbations of the soul or mind, provided a way to take account of the role of the emotions, including grief and sorrow, in the etiology of disease.

## The Passions, Affections, and Emotions:  From A Theory to a Clinical Disease

"Emotion", the more usual English term in recent times, has commonly been defined as an experience characterized by a distinctive feeling or tone (such as love, hate, fear, disgust, anger, joy, or sadness) and some disposition to motor expression. [276] Historically the terms "affection" and "passion" were commonly used English terms, with "passion" and "perturbation of the soul" being the terms of the longest standing.[277] These terms have etymological roots in Latin, therefore, terms like "affectiones" and "affectus" became "affections" and later "affects"; "montus anomorim" became "the soul's motions"; and eventually "emotion" and "pertubationes animorum" became "perturbations of the soul." In the development of a clinical description of *melancholia* over the centuries, fear and sadness were usually key features. Consequently these particular emotional states, or passions or "perturbations of the soul" as they were called in earlier times, had the status of symptoms in a disease. However, they also had the status of affects; this led to their having a place in various theories of the passions or emotions over the centuries. Given those contexts, they were usually aspects of someone's philosophical views

---

[276] Ibid. Jackson
[277] Ibid.

on the nature of man, or later, someone's philosophical psychology. Thus, in some of these contexts the passions themselves were thought of as "diseases of the soul."[278] They did not tend to turn up in medical writings among other diseases, but their emergence in philosophical contexts often entailed the use of a medical metaphor with the implication that corrective measures were needed. Additionally, some affects or passions were taken up in religious systems of thought and given the status of sins, and here again it was not uncommon for a medical metaphor to be used. Using these various contexts, we find terms and emotional states that are analogous to the term *melancholia*. Sadness has commonly been a fundamental symptom of *melancholia*; it was frequently one of the basic passions in various theories of the emotions; and tristitia (sadness, sorrow) was once one of the cardinal sins of the Christian Church. Similarly, one comes across sorrow, dejection, grief, despair, etc., and eventually depression. Thus a brief history of theories on emotions or passions is in order here.

According to Gardiner et al., for Plato, excess of pain or pleasure amounted to disease of the soul in the sense that great distress or joy diminished a person's capacity to reason.[279] The irrational aspects of the soul that were the wellsprings of appetite and feeling were located in the abdominal region and in the chest, respectively, and were potential threats to or antagonists of the smooth functioning of the rational soul, which is located in the brain. The passions that derived from these irrational aspects of the soul were given meanings in terms of the bodily conditions associated with them and so were related to physiology and medical thought. Along with these passions were given ethical meanings, thus placing them in philosophers' theories of emotions and providing the grounds for their

---

[278] Ibid. Pg. 15.
[279] Gardiner, H. M.; Metcalf, Ruth Clark; Beebe-Center, John G. *Feelings and Emotion: A History of Theories* (New York: American Book Company, 1937) Pgs. 10-25.

placement in schemes of religious explanations; whereby from the lowest part of the soul (below the midriff) stemmed the various desires and appetites, from the spirited part of the soul (in the chest) came the affections or passions. Here we see the roots of the medieval classification of the concupiscible affections (the desires and appetites) and the irascible affection (the passions). Plato regarded the various passions partly as modifications of pleasure and pain and partly as distinct.[280] From his perspective, joy and hope were categorized as species of pleasure and grief and fear as species of pain (a scheme that suggests the later emergence of fourfold classification of the passions). Furthermore, it is very important to acknowledge that Plato viewed "the intemperance of the passion of love" as "a disease of the soul" and conceived of love as one of the four cardinal forms of madness, for we will intermittently find "love madness" or "love melancholy" among the categories or forms of *melancholia*.

Aristotle enumerated various passions and perceived them as a category partway between faculties or as predisposing susceptibilities to such affective states, which formed habits; the results of the repeated exercise of said affects.[281] In Aristotle's theory, habits were capacities for behavior that had become established. His theory believed that passions and emotions could be brought under conscious control. Moreover, he believed that these were states accompanied by pleasure or pain, even thought of as species of pleasure or pain; but they differed from pleasure and pain in that they were more complex, were "motions of the soul" and not mere complements of a function.[282] He conceived of "somatic passions", which seemed to be the pains of want and the pleasures of replenishment of the appetites, and of

---

[280] Ibid.
[281] Gardiner, H. M. et al. *Feelings and Emotions: A History of Theories* (New York: American Book Company, 1937) Pgs. 26-27.
[282] Ibid. Gardiner

other passions, other pleasures and pains, which are of the soul. In this theory, some passions being defined as pain or perturbations of the soul did not imply that they were not rooted in bodily processes. Some were described as having origins in both a psychological process and the person's physiological processes. For example, anger was defined as a propensity toward retaliation and as an ebullition of the blood around the heart. The passions were ways in which the soul was affected and were akin to what we call emotions. After Aristotle, the emphasis in the studies of the passions was primarily in the direction of the ethical concerns, including religious concerns. Later came Epicurus, for whom the study of the passions is associated with a doctrine of pleasure; his views were a far cry for any sort of hedonistic orientation.[283] He explicitly dissociated himself from hedonistic ways, indicating that by pleasure he meant the absence of pain in the body, intemperate desire, and all disturbing affections of the soul's imperturbability became the basic good.[284] Thus many of the passions, and particularly extreme forms of the passions, were frowned upon. One was to evade whatever might lead to the greater tumults in the soul.

In contrast to the Aristotelian orientation that the passions should be controlled, the Stoics thought that they should be done away with.[285] Except in the case of the wise man, they viewed them as perverted judgments. They sought inner peace as the basic good and thought of the passions as disorders of the soul, disturbing to reason and contrary to nature. The passions were now defined as "diseases of the soul analogous to those of the body" and thought to be distinguishable from one another in both predisposing temperament and the nature of the disease itself. In spite of that, the Stoics allowed for a class of "good affection," grouped under

[283] Ibid. Pgs. 52-59.
[284] Ibid.
[285] Ibid. Pgs. 64-68.

cheerfulness, discreetness, and a virtuous habit of will; these were "species of quiet emotion befitting the wise" in contrast to the turbulent passions. They also recognized two other categories of emotions: "the natural affections arising from kinship, companionship, etc.," which were viewed favorably, and "the physical pleasure and pains as distinguished from the elation or depression of a mind attending them," which were pleasures and pains viewed "as at least necessary." For the Stoics, in addition to the *feeling state,* the passions involved an impulse toward or away from an object and a judgment about the object. In their scheme of things, there were four basic passions: (1) appetite or desire, an irrational inclination toward implying an opinion of impending evil that seems intolerable (2) fear, an irrational inclination toward implying an opinion of impending evil that seems intolerable (3) pleasure or delight or joy, an irrational expansion or elation of mind, implying a recent opinion of a present good, and (4) pain or grief or sadness, an irrational contraction or depression of mind, implying a recent opinion of a present evil. [286] Subsequently, under these four fundamental passions, various Stoics grouped lists of individual affections and emotional dispositions. From the Greco-Roman period to the end of the 17th century, writers tended to follow the Stoics in "seeking to reduce, classify, and logically define and passions".[287] The Stoic tradition served to establish sorrow, sadness, or grief as one of the basic passion. Of special significance for the study of *melancholia,* it contributed to the emerging recognition of the fundamental antithesis of elation and *melancholy.* Like Plato and the Aristotelian writers, the Stoics gave explicit recognition to the physiological roots of the affections. Though those earlier authors had thought in terms of the humors and their qualities when considering the bodily conditions associated with the passions, the Stoics were apt to think in terms of an enervated

---

[286] Jackson, Stanley W. *Melancholia and Depression: From Hippocratic Times to Modern Times* (New Haven: Yale University Press, 1986) Pgs. 17-25.
[287] Ibid.

pneuma as the bodily concomitant of the troubled states of the soul that were the passions. However, some of the stories employed notions of dispositions of temperament expressed in terms of the humoralist's qualities. Principally, the Stoics followed the tradition that held that the passions had their seat in the heart.

For Plotinus in the 3$^{rd}$ century, all the ordinary passions were merely but the soul's consciousness of the affections of its body.[288] Plotinus, like Plato, believed that the liver was the seat of the bodily appetites and the heart of the nobler impulses. For Plotinus, there were certain blindly working activities of the soul that led to a complex of bodily changes. The soul immediately became aware of these perturbations of the body and associated them with the idea of impending evil; and passion reflected this awareness and experience of the soul. Temperaments and states of illness, conceived of in humoral terms, were thought to dispose a person to particular passions. In his further notions that those who were little inclined to indulge their bodily appetites were less disposed to the various passions and that there were sources of good feelings independent of the body, Plotinus subscribed to views that were taken up by The Church Fathers, supported the endeavor of many mystics, and became integral elements of Christian doctrine.

As was the case with the somatic factors associated with mental disorders in the medical conceptions of ancient Greece and Rome, the bodily commotions associated with the passions were conceived of as integral parts of the passions. Similarly, the humors, the qualities, the temperaments, and the pneuma served the ancient theories of the passions as much as they did the ancient theories of diseases. These orientations continued to prevail throughout The Middle Ages, the Renaissance and in the writings of many later authors. Nemesius in the late 4$^{th}$

---

[288] Ibid. Pgs. 18-25.

century was the most significant of the Patristic writers on the affections.[289] He conceived of the soul as being divided into two parts, the rational and the irrational, a view shared by most Patristic and Scholastic authors. The irrational part had two divisions. There was a vegetative faculty that regulated physiological processes such as waste and repair and was not subject to reason. The other was a part that was subject to reason and subdivided into the concupiscible faculty of appetite or desire and irascible faculty of anger, resentment, or resistance to evil. The passions were associated with the concupiscible and irascible faculties and thus with the irrational part of the soul; yet they were subject to reason. Nemesius viewed them as essential elements of a living person; he thought that they were naturally evil but became so only in combination with reason and will. He distinguished the affections of the body from those of the soul; the former were accompanied by pleasure or pain, while the psychic affection entailed a movement of the appetitive faculty or the irascible faculty sensed as an apprehension of good or evil. He also distinguished between passions that were contrary to nature and induced by alien influences and passions that were associated with a normal fulfillment of function. While employing far fewer subtypes in each category than the Stoics, he fundamentally used a version of their system of four basic species of passion. Of special interest to this study is his view that the seat of grief was in the stomach.[290]

In the 4th century, Gregory of Nyssa elaborated a physiological theory to the effect that in joy and other positive affections the vessels conveying the bodily fluids were dilated, and in painful affections such as grief the vessels were

---

[289] Ibid. Pg. 18.
[290] Ibid. Pg. 19.

contracted.[291] Sadness, despair, and fear were considered at that time to be caused by the constriction of the heart and blood vessels caused, in turn, by the black bile, with its cold and dry qualities. In the 5th century, Augustine conceived of the affections as the soul's motions and identified the passions as a subgroup of the affections, as "those perturbing motions of the soul that are contrary to nature".[292] Against the background of a triadic system of faculties (memory, intelligence, and will) he thought that the root of all affections, including the passions, lay in the will, and he did not refer them to a bodily source.

So it is true that for many centuries some form or other of Plato's scheme of a tripartite soul with concupiscible, irascible, and rational aspects continued to predominate. The former two parts of the soul usually had the affections or passions associated with them and were thought to be actually or potentially in conflict with the rational part. The list of basic affections varied in length, though the most common number was four; most often desire and joy, associated with the concupiscible soul, and fear and sorrow, associated with the irascible soul. Medieval ideas on the passions reached their most complex and probably most influential form in the 13th century with the theories of Thomas Aquinas, within which Aristotelian thought was very effectively integrated with the developing intellectual trends of the Latin West.[293] Aquinas conceived of three levels of the soul - vegetative, sensitive, and rational - each with its own powers or capacities. The vegetative level of the soul entailed the powers of nutrition, growth, and reproduction. The sensitive level and the rational level were each subdivided into cognitive powers and appetitive powers. The cognitive powers were associated

---

[291] Ibid. Jackson
[292] Ibid.
[293] Averill, James. R. *Patterns of Psychological Thought: Reading in Historical and Contemporary Text* (Washington: Hemisphere Publishing Corp., 1976) Pgs. 271-301.

THE HISTORY OF CLINICAL DEPRESSION

with the apprehension of knowledge, and the appetitive powers were the basis for each individual's tendency to fulfill themselves or actualize their potential. For the sensitive level of the soul, the cognitive powers denote five exterior senses (touch, taste, smell, hearing, sight) and four interior senses (common sense, imagination, memory, the estimative power) and the appetitive powers denote the concupiscible and the irascible passions. For the rational level of the soul, the cognitive powers were active and passive reason and the appetitive power referred to the function of the will. In the conception of the "concupiscible" and "irascible" powers as the appetitive powers associated with the sensitive level of the soul (which were often employed by the philosophers of the day) Aquinas was using notions akin to Plato's concupiscible and irascible aspects of the soul. In each case these terms referred to concepts that were key features in the author's theory of the passions. For Aquinas, the concupiscible and irascible powers were tendencies toward objects apprehended intuitively by the exterior and interior senses as either good or evil, and the intensity of such tendencies was the source of the passions. As concupiscible passions, he classified together love, desire, joy, hate, aversion, and sorrow; as the irascible passions he bracketed together hope, despair, courage, fear, and anger. Regarding the relationship of the passions to bodily processes, Aquinas saw the physical changes as vital accompaniments of the affective states but not as causes of these states.

Along with these various theological and philosophical perspectives on the passions, the medical thought of the medieval era involved two important viewpoints on these states. On the one hand, there was the doctrine of the six non-naturals - air, sleep and wakefulness, food and drink, exercise and rest, evacuation and retention, and the passions - that had long provided a framework in which the passions could be viewed as the causes of various somatic effects; and so grief and sorrow could cause bodily ailments. On the other hand, during those same centuries the humoral theory allowed the view that the humors - that is, somatic factors - were causes which could produce affective states as results; the black bile could cause the sadness and fear that were key symptoms in *melancholia*. During the Renaissance there was a significant increase in the amount of writing about the passions, and gradually the affective life came to be viewed in ways somewhat less dependent on theological considerations.[294] The term "affect" and its equivalents were increasingly used, while some began to reserve the terms "passion" and "perturbation" for the more violent affects or the more severe troubling of the soul. Physiological explanations of affective states were increasingly employed once again, with the most common being some notion of the spirits drawn from the traditional doctrine of the pneuma, although the humors and qualities of the humoral theory were still prominent. In conjunction with the humors, affects brought about alterations in the body; and in conjunction with the spirits, they affected the imagination and reason. The distinction between concupiscible and irascible was gradually dropped as the central categorizing principle for affects. Instead, in various classifications there were often two main groupings: those associated with striving for or attaining the good and those associated with avoiding or resisting evil; this system reflected the organizing principles reminiscent of Aquinas's views. Good in the present was associated with pleasure or joy, and evil in the present with pain or sadness. An anticipation of good in the future was associated with desire, and anticipation of evil with fear. A common scheme was a set of primary passions, each of which had associated with it a number of secondary affective states. Some classificatory systems were organized around pleasure and pain as the two primary passions, some were organized by joy

---

[294] Jackson, Stanley, W. *Melancholia and Depression: From Hippocratic Times to Modern Times* (New Haven: Yale University Press, 1986) Pgs. 19-25.

and sadness, and still others were constructed around a set of four primary passions. Quadripartite systems were common, with the terminology varying somewhat - joy (or delight, or pleasure) sadness (or grief, or pain) desire, and fear. Thus sadness, sorrow, or grief was usually one of the basic passions.

The 16th century also saw the first evidence of a change in the longstanding view that the heart was the principal seat of the affects, a trend that was to eventuate in the neurocentric suggestions of the 17th and 18th centuries. Perhaps the best known of these neurocentric theories was that of Descartes. He reaffirmed the tradition of physiological explanation for the passions, using the animal spirits of the nervous system as a key factor and introducing mechanical explanations in place of the line familiar humoral notions.[295] The passions were conceived of as perceptions of affective states by the soul and as caused by movements of the animal spirits that agitated the brain and sustained the impression. With Descartes' dualistic view of soul and body, it was these animal spirits of the nervous system that mediated the interaction between the soul and body. These animal spirits of the nervous system mediated the interaction between the soul and body, particularly through the pineal gland. While the passions were caused by physiological factors, they were of the soul, experienced by the soul. As for what we might term the somatic aspects of an affect, he thought of them merely as accompaniment or effects rather than essential elements. With his concept of neural causation, both the bodily aspects and the felt emotion were effects derived from the same basic somatic cause. He thought of joy and sorrow as the first passions in a person's experience, and he developed a system of six primary passions: admiration (astonishment or surprise) love, hate, desire, joy, and sorrow. In addition to Descartes' important role in the trend toward

---

[295] Cohen, Henry. *The Evolution of the Concept of Disease in Concepts of Medicine: A Collection of Essays on Aspects of Medicine*, ed. Brandon Lush (Oxford: Pergamon Press, 1961) Pgs.159-169.

a neurocentric explanation, his views on the passions were significant in other ways. Although it was by no means new to conceive of the passions as caused by somatic processes, prior to Descartes the Christian Church's ideology had influenced many to think of the affective experience as caused by or stemming from the soul or mind, with its bodily features thus secondary to the passion as felt. He became a principal influence in favor of somatic factors as the root causes of the passions. Further, prior to Descartes the predominant trend in theories of affects had favored the Stoic view that the passions should be subdued rather than expressed, that tranquility was the preferred state. On balance, this view had been favored over the Aristotelian perspective that the passions could be useful spurs toward action. Descartes' *les passions de l'ame* contributed to a shift away the Stoic orientation.

A significant 17th century theorist on the passions was Hobbes, who gave the passions a central place in his considerations of human nature. He viewed them as the guide to thought and the wellspring of action, a constituent of the will, and a determinant of both intellectual and moral tendencies.[296] Hobbes held more to the traditional cardiocentric notion; thinking of the spirits in the region of the heart as the key somatic factors. From basic roots in either appetite or aversion, he developed his set of simple or primary passions: appetite, desire, love, aversion, joy, and grief. Notwithstanding it was far from new to think of the passions as appetitive, as reflecting strivings or desires, Spinoza, also in the 17th century, simplified this orientation to the single basic striving of self-preservation.[297] This theory perpetuated the idea of three primary passions - desire, pleasure, and pain. This simplification plausibly combines the classical representation of them in all

---

[296] Ibid. Pgs. 183-192. Cohen
[297] Ibid. Pgs. 192-205.

systems which operate mainly with logical definitions, where they invariably appear either as forms of conation or as forms of pleasure and pain.[298]

In the 18th century, "affections" and "passions" continued to be frequently used as synonyms.[299] Where they were differentiated, the latter usually referred to more violent or turbulent states. The terms commonly meant the actions or modifications of the mind that followed on the perception of an object or an event usually conceived of as good or evil. Following the Lockean tradition, various sensationalist systems conceived of the passions as being gradually built up from sensations with associationist principles determining the complex of ideas that went to make up a particular passion. Sets of basic passions were postulated; frequently good and evil, respectively, and along with factors of certainty or uncertainty these determined the groupings of both the primary passions and the secondary or compound passions. Some viewed the more violent passions as temporary or if they persisted, as chronic forms of madness. During the latter part of the 18th century, affects were increasingly given a central and fundamental place in the consideration of mental life. This gradually led to assigning the affects an importance that approximated that of intellect. Viewed less in terms of traditional rationalism and conventional morality, the passions came to be extolled as the great impelling forces of human nature.[300] Particularly through the influence of a series of German authors in the late 18th and early 19th centuries, the status of the affects gradually shifted so that a distinct faculty of feeling or affect joined understanding (knowing or cognition) and will (striving or appetition) in a new tripartite system

---

[298] Ibid. Pgs. 197-198. Jackson
[299] Ibid. Pgs. 210-247.
[300] Ibid. Pgs. 247-248.

of faculties.[301] In contrast to the medieval tendency to connect the passions with appetition or desire and to post-Cartesian views that often connected them more with cognition, they came to be thought of as being "as distinct and unique an aspect of mental life as knowing or striving."[302] In summary, during the 18th century the study of "the affects" is still being made by philosophers and the subject matter is treated generally from a vantage point of logic. The psychological aspects of feeling due to more conscientiousness and use of introspection changed the emphasis in studying the disease. Additionally, the new knowledge of the nervous system was used in challenging the theories of dualism and parallelism at the same medical period. Thus, the interest in the feelings has remained keenly alive and a desire to consider them for their own sake foreshadows the coming outgrowth of psychology from philosophy.

Therefore reviewing the 19th century trends in theories of affect, Beebe-Center divided them into peripheral and central theories.[303] By "peripheral" he meant those views that grew out of the sensationalism of the 18th century which emphasized the place of sense organs and physiological processes. Furthermore, by "central" he meant those views that emphasized higher mental processes and sought to explain affects in terms of mental entities. Moreover, in both cases, the theory commonly began with the conscious affective state and then looked in one of these two directions for the factors that were thought to have brought it into being. To the peripheral physiological factors some theories added central notions, but with a somatic emphasis. Often with peripheral physiological factors notions involved the cerebrum, other times other intracranial structures. Other theories of

<hr/>

[301] Jackson, Stanley. W. *Melancholia and Depression: From Hippocratic Times to Modern Times* (New Haven: Yale University Press, 1986) Pgs. 22-25.
[302] Ibid.
[303] Ibid. Jackson

somatic explanation were primarily associated with the central nervous system. Whereas some of the other various physiological theories viewed the subjective states as conscious perception of the somatic process, others thought of them as the end result of these processes and still considered them to be merely additional symptoms.

These reflections of a physiological explanation eventually led to the well-known explanation of the James-Lange theory of emotions. Noting that there had been a tendency for many to think that "the mental perception of some fact excites the mental affection called the emotion, and that this latter state of mind gives rise to the bodily expression", James-Lange went on to say that, on contrary, the "bodily changes follow directly the perception of the exciting fact, and that our feeling of same changes as they occur is the emotion".[304] Given that *melancholia* and *depression* are basic to this study, it is of interest to note that James-Lange concluded that vital bodily features for both sorrow and fear were "weakening of voluntary innervation" and "vasoconstriction" and that joy and elation were associated with an increase of voluntary themes; as sadness, fear, and *melancholy* had recurrently been associated with ideas such as contraction of the mind, constriction of the heart and blood vessels, weakness of the nerves, low nerve energy, low nervous pressure, and constriction of the nerves, and joy and elation had recurrently been associated with ideas such as expansion of the mind, dilation of the heart and blood vessels, excessive nervous pressure, and dilation of the nerves.[305]

The 19th century brought its own theories, which concluded that the disease

---

[304] Ibid.
[305] Ibid. Jackson

started with a mental condition but resulted in an affective state with bodily changes. But as the century went on there was a steady decrease in such fundamental theories of affects or emotions. Physiological explanations became increasingly important, and gradually the focus of such explanations shifted from peripheral organic structures such as the sense organs to central structures of the nervous system. Affects or emotions came to be commonly viewed as attitudes toward objects that involved bodily changes and only secondarily entailed subjective states. By the beginning of the 20th century, Emil Kraepelin's views on *melancholia* and *depression* were in ascendancy. He built his therapeutic program with the "rest cure" as its foundation. He emphasized the removal of the patient from the context in which he had taken ill to an asylum in severe cases and "to a different boarding place or into the association of a happy family" in milder cases. The details of his program included bed rest, constant care, and nutritious diet in small amounts at frequent intervals, warm baths rather than sedatives for insomnia, and precautions against suicidal inclinations. Hypnotics might even be used if milder measures did not suffice. The "psychical influence" of those in attendance was emphasized, with a "gentle, friendly, and assuring" manner advocated for alleviating distress, modifying the delusions, and relieving the anxiety.[306]

Another very prominent view that is central to the 20th century is Adolf Meyer, who recommended an approach more psychologically focused. He advocated a search of the reactive picture for points of modifiability, for foci for intervention and change. He conceived of treatment as "service in behalf of the patient" but he underscored the importance of the patient as a collaborator in the treatment endeavor. He outlined his own "common sense" version of psychotherapy, characterized by kindly, humane overtones and searching practical use of the

---

[306] Ibid. Pgs. 383-395.

patient's life history and current situation. He gave careful attention to the hospital surroundings and how the patient might fit into the hospital and best served by it. However, Kraepelin and Meyer are the benchmark of most of the writings on the treatment of *melancholia* and *depression* during the first part of the 20th century until the emergence of the shock treatment in the 1930's, which was first instituted through the use of metrazol and later with electricity. Subsequently, psychological treatment measures - psychoanalysis and various psychotherapies - came to be used increasingly, both in inpatient and outpatient settings. More recently, antidepressant medication - monoamine oxidase inhibitors and tricyclic anti-depressants - have entered the scene as valuable therapeutic agents. To treat bipolar affective disorders, lithium has come into frequent use.

Last but not least, Sigmund Freud is the most significant author for the middle and the latter part of the 20th century; he is the originator of psychoanalysis. Of particular influence was his paper *Mourning and Melancholia,* which was discussed as early as 1914, written and revised into its final form in 1915, and finally published in 1917.[307] In this study's immediate background were Freud's earlier views on *melancholia* and *depression* and some important observations by his colleague Karl Abraham. Freud sometimes used the term *melancholia* to refer to the range of clinical conditions that the modern psychiatrist would refer to as *depression,* and at other times he was referring only to what today might be termed *psychotic depression.* He used the term *depression* sometimes as a synonym for *melancholia* in either of the two meanings just cited, but more often as a descriptive term for that particular affective aspect of a person's state of mind, whether pathological or not, that might also be called dejection. Freud introduces the notion of *status nervous* where the tendency of *depression* is believed to have

---

[307] Ibid. Pgs. 219-246.

an affect of lowering self-confidence, such as we find very highly developed and in isolation in *melancholia*. There are further instances of *depression* being used as a descriptive term rather than as a diagnostic term. Freud also introduces the term "neurotics" into the analysis of *depression* as a clinical disease.[308]

So yes; threaded through the centuries of clinical description and explanation are a vast number of figurative expressions aimed at conveying what the experience of being *melancholic* was like or how someone came to be *melancholic* - this is the term we now deem to be *depression*. Several metaphors of particular interest and significance appeared and reappeared in these many accounts of *melancholia*. There is constant metaphorical expression, which suggests that there is no one literal statement that would convey the distress of being in the throes of *depression* although there are at least two metaphors that stand out in the long history of *melancholia*: the first being in a state of darkness; the second being weighed down. (Being in a state of darkness was a notion employed in a metaphorical sense by Galen during early Western history. Galen conveyed in his writings something of what it was like to suffer from *melancholia*.) However objective psychologists have become about *depression* or about a particular depressed person, they still manage to identify new factors in *clinical depression* (or someone else's *depression* defined as clinical or otherwise) in every generation. The fact is this disease is likely to confront us via fellow human beings who have serious needs; who know something about great amounts of personal losses, disappointment, and failures. The people we encounter will also know something about being very sad, dejected, dispirited, and broken. With such type distress being described and prominently displayed within our families and communities, we are at the very malaise of what this book argues vexes too many African-American men; a very,

[308] Ibid. Jackson

very serious mental illness that, over time, we have come to know as *clinical depression.*

# Appendix C – Survey Results

*On the Meaning in Life Survey:*

- ✓ Question *one* (1) THE ANSWERS WERE: **8** men answered with #4, **can't say untrue or false**; **2** men answered with #3, **somewhat untrue**; **4** men answered with #1, **absolutely untrue**; and **3** men answered with #2, **mostly untrue.**

- ✓ Question *two* (2) THE ANSWERS WERE: **6** men answered with #2, **mostly untrue**; **6** men answered with #4, **can't say true or false**; **4** men answered with #7, **absolutely untrue**; and **2** men answered with #6, **mostly untrue.**

- ✓ Question *three* (3) THE ANSWERS WERE: **5** men answered with #4, **can't say true or untrue**; **1** man answered with #2, **mostly untrue**; **4** men answered with # 6, **mostly true**; **6** men answered with #3, **somewhat untrue**; and **2** men answered with #5, **somewhat true.**

- ✓ Question *four* (4) THE ANSWERS WERE: **1** man answered with #1, **absolutely untrue**; **7** men answered with #2, **mostly untrue**; **4** men answered with #6, **mostly true**; **3** men answered with #3 **somewhat untrue**; and **3** men answered with #4, **can't say true or false.**

- ✓ Question *five* (5) THE ANSWERS WERE: **1** man answered with #7, **absolutely untrue**; **4** men answered with #2, **mostly true**, **6** men answered with #3, **somewhat untrue**; **6** men answered with #4, **can't say true or false mostly true**; and **1** man answered with #1, **absolutely untrue.**

- ✓ Question *six* (6) THE ANSWERS WERE: **1** man answered with #5, **somewhat true**; **4** men answered with #3, **somewhat untrue**; **6** men answered with #4, **can't say true or false**; **3** men answered with #2, **mostly untrue.**

## SURVEY RESULTS

✓ Question *seven* (7) THE ANSWERS WERE: 2 men answered with #5, **somewhat true;** 6 men answered with #6, **mostly true;** 4 men answered with #7, **absolutely true;** 5 men answered with #4, **can't say true or false;** and 1 man answered with #2, **mostly untrue.**

✓ Question *eight* (8) THE ANSWERS WERE: 7 men answered with #6, **mostly untrue,** 5 men answered with #7, **absolutely true;** 3 men answered with #4, **can't say true or false;** 2 men answered with #3, **somewhat untrue;** 1 man answered with #1, **absolutely untrue.**

✓ Question *nine* (9) THE ANSWERS WERE: 5 men answered with #4, **can't say true or false;** 7 men answered with #6, **mostly true;** 4 men answered with #3, **somewhat untrue;** 1 man answered with #1, **absolutely untrue;** and 1 man answered with #5, **somewhat true.**

✓ Question *ten* (10) THE ANSWERS WERE: 5 men answered with #6, **mostly untrue;** 6 men answered with #7, **absolutely true;** 3 men answered with #4, **can't say true or false;** 3 men answered with #5 **somewhat true;** and 1 man answered with #2, **mostly untrue.**

# Appendix D - Methodologies & Ministry Event

This is a men's ministry Bible study lesson that was meant to focus on self-esteem and being poor and African-American in the United States. This event took place in order to examine the issue of how the men perceived themselves. The study assumes these events would positively influence the awareness and spirituality of where the men are mentally. This lesson also reinforces the theory that African-American men suffer from undiagnosed clinical depression. The method used in this project includes Bible study description, a profile of the project participants, a summary of surveys and participants, and details of the procedures used.

## The Bible Study

On September 26, 2008 and October 24, 2008 I taught a Bible studies class on Judges 6 and Judges 4. These Bible studies were attended by between twenty-five and thirty men and a representation of all age groups within the church was present in the meetings. After praying for insight to deliver the Bible lessons about clinical depression, I introduced our health professionals to the men (a psychologist, a psychiatrist, and a social worker). In addition to being there to advise, their presence was meant to encourage the men to take advantage of any opportunity to meet people who could assist them in countering clinical depression or low esteem.

The Scripture text is Judges 6: 1-18, with an emphasis on verse 15, wherein it says, "And Gideon said unto him, Oh my Lord, wherewith shall I save Israel? Behold, my family is poor in Manasseh, and I am the least in my father's house."[309] The challenge of the text was to have the men experience a sense of the crisis of poverty and powerlessness that is in the text by identifying the position of Gideon in the text. [310] The second text was Judges 4:1-9, with an emphasis on verse 8, that says, "And Barak said unto her, If thou wilt go with me, then I will go: but if thou wilt not go with me, then I will not go."[311] Then, I wanted to compel the men to do some self-examination on how social factors can make men in particular feel insecure, powerless, and subject them to suffer from clinical depression:

**Lesson #1** - I passed out questions to encourage conversation on the subject. Here are the questions from the text in Judges 6:18:

1. What signs of discouragement and low self-esteem did Gideon exhibit in his conversation with the angel? Who was Gideon's father? What was the history of his family?

2. What was the condition of Gideon's people? How does a man feel living in this type of environment?

3. What is the significance of the history of the people of Gideon and why is that in the story?

4. Gideon wondered if God was still with his people, is that still a relevant question today for African-American people?

5. Why was the affirmation of the Lord so important to Gideon? What has happen in your life that makes you need affirmation, as well?

6. Why was it so important for Gideon to build an altar to the Lord? What in the process indicates his low self-esteem?

7. Gideon saw himself as the lowest in his tribe. When one feels like they are

---

[309] The KJV Bible.
[310] Ibid.
[311] Ibid.

nothing, how are they likely to live their lives?

**Lesson #2** - Here are the questions from the second text, Judges 4:1-9:

1.  What are the conditions of the people of Israel at this time?

2.  What does the Scripture state is the cause of the decline in Israel? Can you see the African-American community in this text?

3.  How the position of Canaan in the text does identify with racism in the United States?

4.  Deborah is a prophetess, is she a prophetess because God wanted her, or is she a prophetess because of the lack of leadership within the men? How does her position speak to the condition of women in the African-American community?

5.  Barak's statement says what about him? Why is he so unsure of himself?

6.  Is it alright for men to be vulnerable to women? Why or why not?

7.  What are the benefits of working in tandem with women?

8.  What are the disadvantages of not working with the women?

9.  How does faith benefit men?

10. Comparing the two texts, how are these two men similar?

### During the Class and After

I could sense the men were engaged by the biblical text. Throughout the two classes many men couldn't wait to respond to the questions that were given to them. Moreover, many of the men asked additional questions that were both insightful and reflective on the condition of African-American men in urban areas. One could easily observe that the text and the questions were good for conversation for the men. This is the area in the conversation where the invited therapist and social worker were helpful; they contributed data and demographics on how mental health is vitally important to the African-American community.

It's important to hold these sessions/Bible studies to just one hour and a half or so. Furthermore, the leader of the class session should encourage the men to not be judgmental or arrogant during conversations so that there will be more time for conversational interaction. The teacher/facilitator should not be doing all the talking during the class session. I would also encourage all the participating men and young men to sit down in this conversational setting rather than standing up; this seems to create more of an environment for sharing and community during the discussion. Additionally, I would encourage the teacher/facilitator to stay longer afterwards and allow men to approach. In my observation, many men share individually afterwards in these kinds of forums, and relish the chance to speak to one another in a one on one situation. I noticed that after each class men would sit around and want to talk longer, and though I insisted that we conclude on time, many men wanted to stay after the meeting and talk on specific events and personal struggles within their lives as well. Therefore, I strongly encourage the teacher/facilitator to include time for the men to talk after the meeting and allow the health professionals and social workers to bring and disseminate their cards for the men to contact them later, if they so desire.

After doing this a few times, I noticed that each class session began to become larger and larger. I believe the men were enlightened and inspired while being made aware of possibilities concerning their mental health, especially with respect to clinical depression. And the feedback from the men has definitely been encouraging on the subject; the positive responses actually superseded what I believed would be the general reception of discussing the topic of clinical depression. The classes also allowed me to challenge the men to do the things that are listed in this book to help maintain their good mental health.

In conclusion, I believe pastors should constantly lift the themes and topics in Scripture that allow him or her to deal with the subject of clinical depression in sermons, Bible lessons, and small groups. I would also encourage pastors to look at various passages in Scripture from the perspective of a clinically depressed person, so that people are aware of how the symptoms of clinical depression can impact one's choices, personality, and lifestyle. Due to the pervasiveness of clinical depression, the pastor and the church's leadership should do all it can to encourage people to be as mentally healthy as possible. We know that in the African-American tradition especially, it is often easier to get people to act after hearing a sermon than at any other time. Thus, sermons that address mental health or clinical depression should be insightful, provocative, and non-judgmental. I encourage that, when possible, whenever one heavily preaches on such a theme to have a mental health care professional or social worker there for conversation immediately afterwards. Always remember that how you, as the leader, engage the topic will help to determine how the people perceive and accept the information.

# BIBLIOGRAPHY

Akbar, Na'im. *Breaking the Chains of Psychological Slavery* (Tallahassee: Mind Productions & Associates, 1996).

Averill, James. R. *Patterns of Psychological Thought: Reading in Historical and Contemporary Text* (Washington: Hemisphere Publishing Corp., 1976).

Bakari, Kitwana. *Young Blacks and the Crisis in African -American Culture: The Hip Hop Generation* (New York: Perseus Books Group, 2002).

Blackmon, Douglas. A. *Slavery by Another Name: The Re-Enslavement of Black Americans from the Civil War to World War II* (New York: Double Day Broadway Publishing Group, 2008).

Blount, Brian K.; Cain Hope Felder; Clarice J. Martin; Emerson B. Powery, Associate Editors. *True to Our Native Land: An African-American New Testament Commentary* (Minneapolis: Fortress Press, 2007).

Boothe, Demico. *Why Are So Many Black Men In Prison?* (Memphis: Full Surface Publishing, 2007).

Cohen, Henry. *The Evolution of the Concept of Disease in Concepts of Medicine: A Collection of Essays on Aspects of Medicine* (Oxford: Pergamon Press, 1961).

Cone, James H. *God of the Oppressed* (New York: Seabury Press, 1975).

Du Bois, W.E.B. *The Souls of Black Folk* (New York: Penguin Books, 2003 {1903}).

Edge, Findley B. *A Quest for Vitality in Religion* (Nashville, Tennessee: Broadman Press, 1963).

Evans, Jr., James H. *We Shall All Be Changed* (Minneapolis: Fortress Press, 1997).

Gardiner, H. M. et al. *Feelings and Emotions: A History of Theories* (New York: American Book Company, 1937).

Gibbs, Jewelle. et. al. *Young Black and Male in America: An Endangered Species* (Dover: Auburn House Publishing Company).

Gilbert, Paul. *Overcoming Depression: Step-By-Step to Gaining Control Over Depression 2nd Ed.* (New York: Oxford Press, 1997).

Gillette, Howard. *Camden After the Fall: Decline and Renewal in a Post-Industrial City* (Philadelphia: University Of Pennsylvania Press, 2005).

Griesinger, Wilhelm. *Die Pathologie und Therapie der psychisen Krankbeiten* (Stuttgart: Adolph Krabbe, 1845 newer translation 1972).

Jackson, Stanley W. *Melancholia and Depression: From Hippocratic Times to Modern Time* (New Haven: Connecticut, 1986).

# BIBLIOGRAPHY

Kelsey, David H. *Between Athens and Berlin: The Theological Education Debate* (Grand Rapids: William Erdmann Publishing Company, 1993).

Klibansky, Raymond; Erwin Panofsky; and Fritz Saxl. *Saturn and Melancholy: Studies in the History of Natural Philosophy, Religion and Art* (New York: Basic Books, 1964).

Kouzes, James M. and Barry Z. Posner. *The Leadership Challenge* (San Francisco: Jossey-Bass, Publisher, 2003).

Kunjufu, Jawanza. *State of Emergency: We Must Save African-American Males* (Chicago: African-American Images, 2001).

Leary, Joy Degruy. *Post Traumatic Slave: America's Legacy of Enduring Injury and Healing* (Milwaukee: Uptone Press, 2005).

Lincoln, C. Eric. *Black Church: Christianity and Crisis,* vol. 30, No. 18 (1970).

Louis, Uchitelle. *The Disposable Worker: Layoffs and Their Consequences* (New York: Vintage Books 2007).

Meyer, Adolf. *The Collected Papers of Adolf Meyer, ed. Eunice E. Winters, 4 vols.* (Baltimore: The John Hopkins Press, 1951).

Real, Terrence. *I Do Not Want To Talk About It: Overcoming The Secret Legacy Of Male Depression* (New York: Scribner, 1997).

Roberts, J. Deotis. *The Roots of a Black Future: Family and Church* (Philadelphia, PA: Westminster Press, 1980).

Salley, Columbus and Ronald Behm. *What Color Is Your God?* (Downers Grove, Illinois: Intervarsity Press, 1981).

Sigerist, Henry E. *A History of Medicine, 2 vols.* (New York: Oxford University Press, 1951-1961).

The Holy Bible, the King James Version.

Thompson, Rondel. *The State of Black America 2006* (New York: National Urban League Press, 2006).

Wallis, Jim. *God's Politics: A New Vision for Faith and Politics in America* (New York: HarperCollins Publishers, 2005).

Weems, Jr., Lovett H. *Church Leadership Vision, Team, and Integrity* (Nashville, TN: Abingdon Press, 1993).

West, Cornel. *Race Matters* (Boston: Beacon Press, 1993).

Williams, Terrie M. *Black Pain: It Just Looks Like We're Not Hurting* (New York: Scribner Books, 2008).

Wilson, William Julius. *When Work Disappears: The World of the New Urban Poor* (New York: Vintage Books, 1996).

CPSIA information can be obtained at www.ICGtesting.com
Printed in the USA
BVOW032051210312

285712BV00005B/312/P